THE RUNNING REVOLUTION

"The Pose Method of running has not only eliminated my injuries, it has been an integral part of continued improvement in my chosen sport. In fact at fifty-two years of age I am still improving. A bonus of the Pose Method for me has been significant health and strength improvement. My journey has been patient and progressive and had I continued to run as I did previously I believe I would now be limited to playing board games. My advice is to be patient and persevere; it truly is worth it."

> —Terry Roberts, twenty-eight time Ironman finisher and
> Ironman Australia legend

"I have used these principles to develop running skill in U.S. Army Soldiers since 2008 and have seen decreases of up to four minutes on a two-mile run within just two weeks."

> —Dr. Charles Blake, U.S. Army Major and physical therapist

"About one year ago, I could not run fifty yards without extreme IT Band Syndrome pain. I spent thirty minutes with Dr. Romanov and could run as far and as much as I wanted pain free. Today, I am the USA Paratriathlon National Champion."

> —David Kyle, associate director of health and physical education,
> University of Alabama

"The material and insights detailed in *The Running Revolution* are scientifically, physically, and emotionally profound. The Pose Method has the potential to be used as a standard by which running performances can be evaluated, coached, and enhanced. If you are a runner looking for a resource to reduce injury risk, improve performance, and build your training program, look no further. In twenty-five years of working with running athletes, I have yet to find a more meaningful resource."

> —Tom Whipple, physical therapist, Penn State Sports Medicine,
> and author of *The Endurance Paradox*

"Romanov's teachings have dramatically changed and fundamentally shaped the way we think about, understand, and teach not only running, but all movement. I can say unequivocally that no other information I have acquired in my career has influenced my teaching process more. The Pose Method is the only teaching method we use for our runners at La Palestra."

> —Pat Manocchia, former *Good Morning America* fitness expert and
> founder of La Palestra Center for Preventative Medicine

"To tens of thousands of runners, including me, Nicholas Romanov walks (and runs) on water. Approaching running as a skill to be learned, his groundbreaking, much-copied Pose Method established a new paradigm, promoting a soft, natural landing that minimizes impact, maximizes speed, eliminates injuries, and saves running careers. No one thought about form until Romanov came along; now we know that it is crucial. I've interviewed dozens of runners who simply would not be running without it."

—Roy M. Wallack, author of *Barefoot Running Step by Step* and *Run for Life*

"The Pose Method of running has been a crucial component of my physical therapy practice. Not only does this method offer a clear standard for teaching and modifying running form, it also allows runners to run more efficiently. I instruct my patients in the Pose Method before allowing them to run again. Since adopting this practice I have seen patients who were unable to run for years not only start running again, but do so pain free. Other patients have shaved one to two minutes, on average, off their two-mile Army Physical Fitness Test run times. Since learning the Pose Method, I have personally dropped my half marathon time by ten minutes."

—Major Angela Diebal, U.S. Army physical therapist

"There's no doubt about it, the Pose Method made me a more efficient runner. And the beauty of the system is that no matter who you are, if you stick to the principles and apply them in each training session, you can't help but improve."

—Andrew Walters, elite Australian Marathoner, Pose Method coach,
and founder of Setai-Do Australia

"I discovered Dr. Romanov's Pose Method about four years ago, and it has changed the way I understand running. Since then both my athletes and I have gained the ability to run great distances with less stress on the body, faster recovery, and reduced running-related injuries. This book will help transform you into a smoother, more confident athlete."

—Gil Cramer, running technique specialist and elite ultra marathoner

"Movement skill is foundational for the performance community. Dr. Romanov brings the same approach to running. Romanov's *Running Revolution* is the common standard upon which running skill can be built."

—Major David Feltwell, U.S. Army physical therapist

"Dr. Romanov has spent the majority of his life thinking about running problems and in close to one day the solutions came to him: Pose Method. I am overwhelmed by gratitude when I ponder how much time Dr. Romanov has invested into solving many of the running problems we have not understood in the past."

—Debbie Savage, strength and conditioning coach,
Australian Sports Commission, and former elite sprinter

PENGUIN BOOKS

THE RUNNING REVOLUTION

DR. NICHOLAS ROMANOV is a two-time Olympic coach and world-renowned sports scientist with a career spanning more than forty years. He has conducted research worldwide, including in the United States, Canada, the United Kingdom, South Africa, and New Zealand. As a former elite record-holding national high jumper, Dr. Romanov created the Pose Method in the 1970s. He founded Romanov Academy in the 1990s to certify and educate coaches teaching sports technique. There are now thousands of Pose Method certified Technique Specialists worldwide. Over the last several decades, the Pose Method has been utilized at an institutional level with large organizations including the United States Military, CrossFit, and professional sports programs including the National Triathlon teams of Great Britain, United States, and Russia. Dr. Romanov also works with medical professionals including physical therapists, podiatrists and orthopedic surgeons. He travels around the world conducting research, consulting professional sports organizations, and as a motivational speaker. Dr. Romanov lives in Miami.

KURT BRUNGARDT has covered the sports and fitness beat for nearly twenty years. He has written ten books on fitness and sports training, including the bestsellers *The Complete Book of Abs* and *The Complete Book of Core Training*. He has written for *Men's Health*, *SLAM*, and *Vanity Fair*. His 2007 feature article for *Vanity Fair*, "Galloping Scared," was nominated for a Genesis Award. Most recently, he covered the 2010, 2011, 2012, and 2013 NBA draft for SLAMonline. He is the creator of the multipart documentary series *Undrafted* for SLAMonline, which started in 2012 and is now in its third year. He's a contributor to Weight Watchers online and is the associate editor for the Web site ProHoopStrength.com (a Web site started by NBA strength coaches). He has also produced and directed exercise videos, most notably the Billboard Top 10 classic *Abs of Steel for Men* as well as *Action Sports Camp* (a workout for kids), hosted by NBA All-Star and champion Sean Elliot. He lives in New York City.

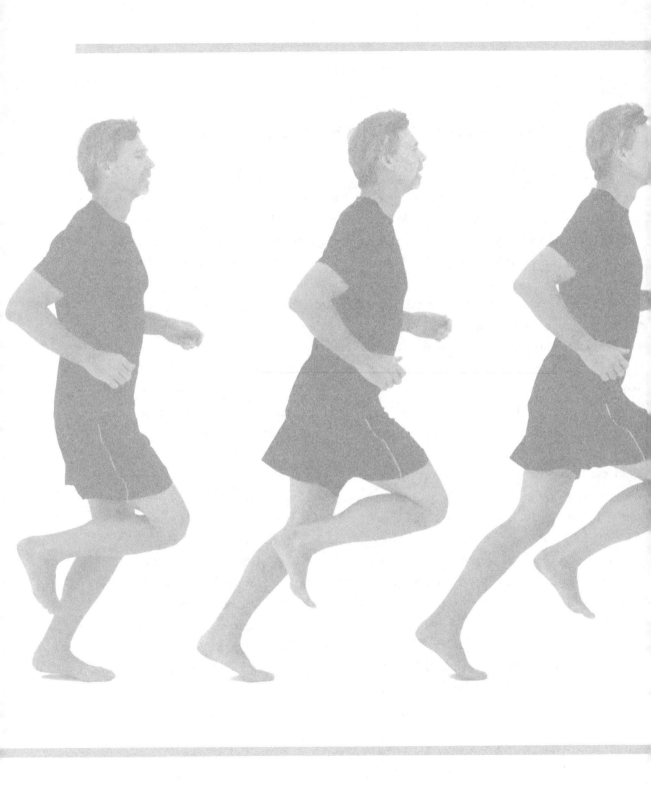

THE RUNNING REVOLUTION

HOW TO RUN FASTER, FARTHER, AND INJURY-FREE—FOR LIFE

DR. NICHOLAS ROMANOV
with KURT BRUNGARDT

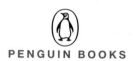

PENGUIN BOOKS

PENGUIN BOOKS

Published by the Penguin Group
Penguin Group (USA) LLC
375 Hudson Street
New York, New York 10014

USA | Canada | UK | Ireland | Australia | New Zealand | India | South Africa | China
penguin.com
A Penguin Random House Company

First published in Penguin Books 2014

Infographics and drawings: Benjamine Reid / Pose Method, Inc.
Photographs: Luis Piñol / Pose Method, Inc.
Shoe sketches on page 30: Andrey Pyanzin / Pose Method, Inc.

ISBN 978-0-14-312319-4

Printed in the United States of America
3   5   7   9   10   8   6   4

Set in Bembo with Helvetica Neue Display
Designed by Elke Sigal

ACKNOWLEDGMENTS

This book would never have come together without the tremendous effort of my family, colleagues, and friends, who provided never-ending support in my journey to bring this knowledge to the world. I am forever grateful to all of them.

The continuous passionate work of my wife Svetlana, the spirit of my daughter Marianna, the creativity of my daughter Lana, the dedicated work of my son Severin, and the heartwarming support of my son Nicky and granddaughter Sophia have always been the main driving forces behind my work.

I can't express enough how much I appreciate my pleasant collaboration with Kurt Brungardt, whose talent helped me to express all these ideas in an easy-to-read free flowing manner. My sincere thank you to my dear friend and colleague Dr. Graham Fletcher, whose efforts and dedication to provide a scientific background for the Pose Method are priceless. Many thanks to Ben Reid for his creative work on developing the images and illustrations for this book and to our steady-handed photographer Luis Piñol.

Thank you to our friends Nicole Vassilaros, Chris Drozd, Ed Bugarin, Carol Jaxon, and Eike Schwartz for their tireless work in the studio as the best fitness models anyone could ask for.

I am grateful to the army of runners, triathletes, and fitness enthusiasts around the world who have accepted the Pose Method as their way of running, which continues to be my inspiration to continue perfecting my work.

DR. NICHOLAS ROMANOV

In chronological order: Thanks to Dr. Romanov and his entire family for sharing their homes in Miami for extended stays, when we worked on the book. Also, thanks to Dr. R and Severin for patiently sharing their knowledge. Thanks to Dan Strone and Trident Media for having confidence in the book. I'd also like to thank my brothers, who are always helpful in conversation and advice in the areas of sports and fitness. And, of course, as always, my mother for her humor, interest, and support.

Thank you to everyone at Penguin, the editors, production staff, and marketing team for bringing this book to readers. Specifically, we'd like to thank our fantastic editors; this process started with Tara Singh Carlson, then moved on to Liz Van Hoose. Liz handed it off to Ramona Demme, who eventually handed it back to Tara for the last stages—true teamwork. Thank you to senior publicist Meredith Burks for her work, and finally editor in chief Patrick Nolan for his support of this project.

KURT BRUNGARDT

To my son Severin, with my love and sincere appreciation of his tremendous dedication and efforts that made this book possible —N.R.

To Tracy Marx (sometimes Karl, sometimes Groucho), who is always a willing partner in a revolution. —K.B.

CONTENTS

PART ONE
PREPARING FOR THE POSE

PART TWO
TEN LESSONS

PART THREE
THE RUNNING CIRCUIT

PART FOUR
TAKE IT TO THE LIMIT

INTRODUCTION

How to Run Like the Best in the World

Here's a breakdown of Usain Bolt's world record 100-meter race in Berlin in 2009: 9.58 seconds. Forty-one steps. Time on the ground—3.20 seconds. Time in the air—6.38 seconds. Running is flying.

If you watch it on YouTube, adding to the thirteen million–plus views, a feeling of wonder might surprisingly well up inside you. It's like seeing any great performance in sports or the arts; it takes you somewhere beyond. To see a human run that fast—faster than any other human on the planet has ever run (at least in modern history)—triggers something deep in the body about our movement potential, about our ability to master our mind-body relationship in an essential way, erasing perceived limits.

Bolt doesn't want to stop when he crosses the finish line. He gears down but he keeps running, and even as he coasts across space, you won't be able to take your eyes off him. Maybe it's because his movements are an inseparable bond of beauty and efficiency. Or maybe you stare with a coach's eye, hoping that in a flash something will be revealed, some secret— Oh, *now* I see how he does it. He spreads his arms like wings, because he was flying.

Whether he knows it not, Bolt is a poster child for the Pose Method. Bolt is an athletic genius, just like Bach, Mozart, and Beethoven were musical geniuses. He tapped into nature's blueprint for running, and to analyze his technique reveals how nature designed us to run optimally. The techniques you will learn in *The Running Revolution* were discovered by watching how the best runners in the world run (more on this in the next chapter).

There are other Pose poster runners. When Michael Johnson electrified the world with his gold medal performances in the 200- and 400-meter runs at the 1996 Olympics in Atlanta, television analysts and sports writers made numerous references to his short, choppy strides and his erect running stance. It was clear watching video replays that Johnson's technique was utterly different from all of his competitors, who all had longer strides and more of a forward bend at the waist. The commentators mentioned the difference but never really seemed to analyze it.

At the other end of the distance spectrum, another Olympic champion and a world record holder at the 5K and 10K distances, Haile Gebrselassie, told *Running Times* magazine how his technique was formed. "When I was fourteen or fifteen," he said, "I remember my brother tried to encourage me by giving me a pair of running shoes. But I threw them away, because I was used to running with bare feet, and the shoes were too heavy." Running without shoes is one of the best ways to get in touch with nature's blueprint. What makes this interesting is that these two runners, arguably the greatest sprinter and distance runner, respectively, in history share an almost identical technique.

Johnson lands on the ball of his foot. And those short, choppy strides, which captivated the Olympic viewing audience, indicate the rapid turnover (change of support legs), propelling him to a breathtaking time of 19.32 seconds in the Olympic 200-meter race, quite possibly the greatest single run in history. Yet if you were to approach either Johnson or Gebrselassie and say, "I see you use the Pose Method of running," they would not have the slightest idea what you were talking about.

Now you may be asking: What does this have to do with me? Are you going to help me set a world record? If you are someone who runs for health, fitness, and occasionally runs races, the answer is no. But completing the lessons and program in this book will improve your running technique, decrease your chances of injury, and help you set a personal record. If you are an elite world-class runner, then yes, this book may help you set a world record. The technique is the same for all speeds of running, from an all-out sprint to a slow jog. For both the elite and the recreational runner, if you follow the program, the promise is the same:

- You will run more efficiently.
- You will run faster.
- You will be able to run greater distances while maintaining the optimal form.
- You will decrease your chances of injury.

HOW THE BODY WAS DESIGNED TO RUN

In the past, among amateurs and professionals alike, the consensus was that everyone has their own unique way of running, and there's no right or wrong technique. To take arms against this notion is to invite an attack that would make grown men cry.

Nonetheless, the manifesto statement of *The Running Revolution* is just that: There is a universal, archetypical running form. Nature gives us a blueprint—a blueprint that, to the detriment of runners everywhere, has been largely ignored. The result: About two-thirds of runners are injured every year—a figure that would be considered unacceptable in any other sports activity.

Cue the opening of *Anna Karenina.* "All happy families are alike; each unhappy family is unhappy in its own way." You could say the same thing about running. All happy runners are alike (they adhere to the universal standard), but all unhappy runners are unhappy in their own way (unique and varied deviations from the standard). Okay, it was a stretch to sneak in Tolstoy, but you see the point. The Pose Method at the heart of this book will restore your focus to the universal standard of running you were born with.

In a nutshell, this book, supported by the latest research, is a detailed and practical answer to the question: Is there one universal, correct way to run? It's not a dissertation on whether or not we were born to run. Chris McDougall, in his bestselling book *Born to Run,* answered this question for the mass audience. This is not a book about your running physiology, developing your cardiovascular system, staying in target heart-rate zones, or programming a training schedule based on miles and times. It's also not about your diet. It's not yoga for runners, or Pilates for runners, or weight training for runners. The shelves are packed with these books.

What the shelves aren't filled with are books that actually teach you *how* to run. That's what this book is about. It's about running technique, optimal biomechanics, and skills and drills to improve your running form. Really, that's all there is. Everything else is secondary. If your technique sucks (pardon the Russian), you're not addressing the core issues of improving your speed, endurance, efficiency, or running economy. It's no longer a debate that running, and the way we think about running, is changing fast. We are now on the other side of the paradigm shift. These rules are new to the degree that you were taught to run with a heel strike or you were told that everyone has their own unique running technique. Once again, shoe design, with the minimalist trend (now a multibillion-dollar segment of the market) has been the driving force in this sea-change approach to running form. Now mainstream runners are asking variations on the questions I first raised nearly forty years ago: Is landing on my heel first the wrong way to run? (Yes.) Am I supposed to land on my forefoot? (Yes.) Should I run barefoot? (Not necessarily.)

This book will help you navigate the maze, cutting through all the confusion.

RUNNING IS A SKILL

To consider something a skill, you have to believe there is a right and wrong way to do it, a standard and a deviation. The right way—the standard—can be taught and developed. Since running form has been thought of as something intrinsic and unique to each individual, it has not been taught with any detail, except to elite athletes. You might be wondering how the natural way to run—the way we were born to run—came to be a skill that now has to be taught. The long and the short of it is that the modern sneaker, with its built-up heel and motion control support, enables poor technique: heel striking, muscle atrophy, limited sensory feedback from the feet, and more. We have been running incorrectly for so long that it's no longer natural for us to run the way nature intended. We must relearn how to run.

RUNNING IS AN ATHLETIC EVENT

You are an athlete. You will be treated like an athlete and be expected to behave like a model athlete. Therefore, you will:

- Show up to every lesson on your scheduled plan.
- Stay focused and complete all elements of your lessons.
- Be patient and keep a positive attitude when things get tough or when you don't see immediate results.

This book is designed like a semester-long class. It's a workbook built around ten units, each intended to last a week or more—however long it takes you to internalize the new concepts and gain the strength to execute them. Because learning how to run is a step-by-step process, it will take time for these concepts and new ways of moving to settle into your body and replace old, inefficient patterns.

The best way to wrap your head around this new method is to approach the book as you would a complex recipe: Read it all the way through first to get the big picture, then start with Lesson One and follow the program in order. The information contained in these lessons is cumulative and progressive. Don't get hung up on attaining perfection before moving to the next lesson. Throughout the program you'll be revisiting key techniques to ensure that the tenets of previous lessons are still being upheld.

If ever you need a quick reminder of a particular stretch or strength drill, consult the appendix. You can also visit www.posemethod.com, where you will find a worldwide network of clinics, running groups, and certified coaches who use the Pose Method. Most important, always remember that you are on the path to running faster, longer, and stronger. Your biggest reward will be a lifetime of joyful, injury-free running.

THE
RUNNING
REVOLUTION

PART ONE

PREPARING FOR THE POSE

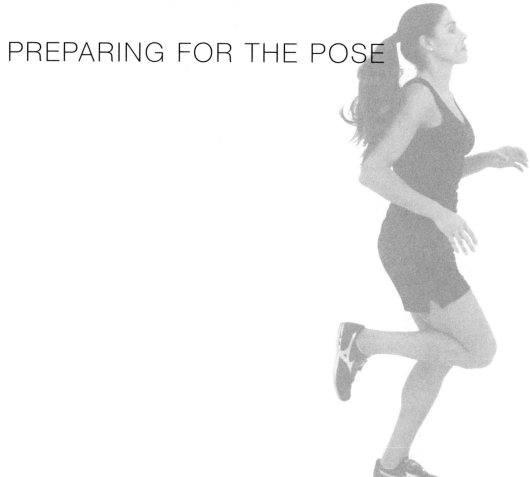

A PERSONAL HISTORY OF RUNNING

My Journey from Russia to America

My crisis began on a cool, rainy October morning in 1977. I was returning home from the sports training facility at my university, the Pedagogical University, located some six hundred kilometers from Moscow in the city of Cheboksary, Russia. The university was a key gear in the Soviet Union's awesome athletic machine. Many of our athletes would go on to score Olympic medals, set world records, and lead powerhouse Soviet teams.

My mood was in tune with the gloomy day, downcast and sullen. I was a teacher of track and field at the Pedagogical University. To American ears this translation sounds funny, like it's missing its name. In Russia, the names of all state-run institutions reflected their function, not their affiliation or location like Harvard or the University of Texas. The Pedagogical University was like the Teachers College of Columbia University, except our specialization was training future coaches, PE teachers, and elite athletes.

I was a recent graduate from the university, and now a track and field coach working on my PhD. As a young scientist and coach, the future seemed bright. But that morning, as I walked home from my track and field lesson on running, my mood was low. I felt incompetent, even after all my hard work.

After all the school's accomplishments, after all the important scientific work done by the prestigious faculty, and after two years of working with students and doing postgraduate studies, I realized I was caught in a paradox. On the one hand, I was now equipped with more facts and knowledge than ever before. I had made the transition from competitive athlete to coach and scientist, yet I realized that all my education and experience had not equipped me to teach my students such a seemingly simple exercise as running.

The problem wasn't that I was a bad student. On the contrary, I had graduated at the top of my class. I had been exposed to pretty much everything about running that had been accumulated in scientific and educational practice at that time. But the one thing I wanted most—a scientifically based method of teaching running technique—was simply nonexistent in the then-current theory and practice. What did exist were generally contradictory viewpoints on running technique and methods of teaching it.

One prevailing theory held that running was second nature to humans and should not or could not be taught, since each individual's running style was preordained, essentially at birth, by his or her physical stature. Another bit of popular wisdom was that the appropriate running technique differed for sprints, middle distances, and marathons and thus required different ways of teaching it in each case. Most qualified coaches and teachers did agree on one thing: running is a simple exercise, and the best runners are those who combine the hardest training with superior genetic makeup.

Following this reasoning, they felt there was little necessity to pay much attention to the specifics of running technique, unlike other track and field events like jumping, hurdling, or throwing, or for that matter, other movement disciplines like ballet, karate, or wrestling, where technique was of paramount importance.

In that dark moment I realized that basically I didn't know what running was from either a biomechanical or a psychological standpoint. Consequently, I couldn't teach it to my students (future coaches and physical education instructors) or my athletes. I felt simultaneously powerless and challenged.

During this walk I had become resolute in my life's quest: unlocking the mystery of the biomechanics of running and finding the best ways to teach it.

I went to work as a student of science. I observed countless hours of footage of the world's best runners. To do this analysis, I looked at filmstrips of them running, frame by frame. What I began to notice was not the differences but a remarkable similarity in technique. Sure, they had stylistic differences, but the best runners were all essentially doing the same thing. The idea came to me in an instant. All movement has a key position that defines it.

Through my investigation, I identified three universal elements that all runners move through. They all passed through what I began to call the key Pose in the dynamic movement of running. I now call these elements the running Pose, falling, and pulling. To my surprise I began to notice that average runners, in fact everyone, cycled through these three elements. In less adept runners it is harder to see, but they were doing the same thing as great runners, just not as efficiently.

I didn't yet understand the function of these three key elements but I knew they were present in every type of running, from the morning jog to the sprint to the ultramarathon. As I said, great runners executed these key elements with great efficiency. I would even say with beauty, grace, and effortlessness. In the not-so-great runners, the transitions between these elements could be downright ugly. They looked heavy and exhibited excessive muscular effort with lots of wasted movement and noise. Great running, I realized, required the mastery of clean, precise movement from the running Pose to falling to pulling and back to the running Pose.

Sometime thereafter, I went back to the Greeks and worked my way forward. I was always attracted to Plato's theory of ideal forms. It reassured me that there could be an ideal form of running.

I found inspiration in Aristotle's early attempts at science and physics, nearly two thousand years before Newton's laws. Aristotle said that which causes movement and that which remains still must be equal. For running, this means you can't move forward without a base of support. This was the antecedent for Newton's great discoveries.

It was also hard to ignore the art of the Greeks. The paintings of runners on the vases depict more than artistic flights of fancy. I believe they are accurate depictions of how the Greeks ran. The drawings illustrate different running speeds, from a sprint to a jog. They also show a similarity of running form, whether sprinting or running long distance. The running movements of the athletes on these vases convinced me that the ancient Greeks observed the key elements of optimal running technique. The paintings show that all the athletes land with their weight on their forefoot.

I worked my way up to the great thinkers of the Renaissance and ran head-on into Leonardo da Vinci. As with almost everything he did, he was way ahead of his time when it came to understanding human movement. His studies, designed to help his students accurately represent motion on the canvas, led him to proclaim that humans always project their weight in the direction of the place they are moving toward—the faster a human runs, the more he leans toward his destination, placing more of his weight in front of his axis of balance than behind it.

Considering Leonardo's other achievements and his place in Western civilization, you would think this would have focused the conversation. His observation targets what I assert to be a key element of running—the falling phase. Running is harnessing the diluted effects of gravity by falling forward.

From the Renaissance, I moved to the Enlightenment and Sir Isaac Newton. It was Newton's Law of Universal Gravitation and his Laws of Motion that ultimately revealed the undeniable force that shapes all motion—including human movement. This focused my work on the effects of gravity as a leading force in running. Many years later my colleague Dr. Graham Fletcher brought to my attention the work of a Scottish mountaineer and physiologist, Thomas Graham-Brown (1882-1965). Applying Newton's ideas to the study of human activity, Brown theorized that when a body runs along the ground, the center of gravity is permitted to fall forward and down under the influence of gravity—the momentum the runner's body achieves with gravity is what propels the body forward.

I want to make an important point that is often misunderstood about the Pose method and my work. My discovery of the running Pose, the fall angle, and pulling action in running are not opinions but are observational and conceptual descriptions of optimal running form that are now part of the scientific community. With these findings, I was able to describe how the body was designed to run. The three key elements and the effect of gravity on the way we run are the subjects of my work as a scientist.

I didn't invent a new way of running; the Pose Method just describes how the body is designed to run. I'm naming and teaching what is a natural process, but a process that has become perverted by harmful shoes and poor coaching. However, if you've ever heard seemingly random tips for running like "don't overstride," or "shorten your stride," or "lean" into the run, there is a good chance those tips were influenced by the Pose Method and my research.

I also can't claim that every world-class runner moves in perfect alignment with nature's blueprint. The very best are close to this standard, which is an ideal, like Plato's forms. Some great runners, because of their genetic gifts, have many deviations and still win. Coaching, drills, and the most effective strength training methods for running would bring them closer to the standard and make them even better.

Lastly, perfection of the Pose Method does not turn runners into Pose machine clones of one another. Even the best masters of running form will retain their unique stylistic flourishes that are optimal for their individual body type and psychology, just like cars have different styles and bodies but a similar infrastructure. Some car bodies are built for speed, like a Ferarri, others are built for power. Pose Method mastery would not turn Haile Gebrselassie into Usain Bolt.

So, back to my salad days, circa 1977. I'm supposed to be a young hotshot coach at one of Russia's leading universities for sports. The 1970s is the golden age for sports science in Russia and I wanted to leave my mark. I've had my big revelation, I know the elements of running; now I have to confront a basic question head-on as I face my students: What's the best way to teach people to run?

My coaching revelation came through observing how other athletes trained—martial artists, wrestlers, and also ballet dancers. Ballet was particularly easy to study living in Russia where the art and tradition were developed to perfection. I had friends who were ballet dancers, and I was able to watch both their training sessions and performances. My observations of some of the world's greatest ballerinas left me with a burning question: Why is it that the movements in ballet and even karate and wrestling are so perfect? Could it be narrowed down to the number of repetitions of simple exercises? The answer came on as a sudden flash of insight. Simplicity itself is the key.

I realized that training in ballet, martial arts, and wrestling is done as a series of precise poses. Through these poses and drills, the perfection of movement is achieved and integrated into a flow. Everything fell into place for me immediately, like the pieces of a puzzle.

Then I faced a fundamental question: What is the precise pose and drills that apply to running? The logical answer was the universal positions and actions that all runners do—the three elements I'd isolated and named after watching all that running footage: *the running Pose*, *falling*-forward, and *pulling* the support foot off the ground.

But even as I developed a deeper understanding of these elements, my conclusions, although backed by science, were not accepted by the running community because they went against the traditional paradigm. Coaches, sports scientists, and

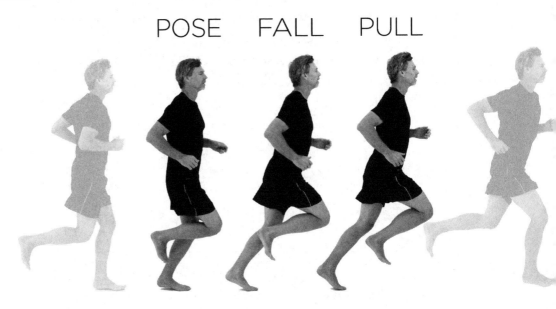

POSE   FALL   PULL

The three foundational elements in running

runners largely followed a model created in England in the 1960s by Geoffrey Dyson in the *Mechanics of Athletics*. Dyson defined support, drive, and recovery as the three phases of running. For decades in the running world, the Pose Method was not universally accepted.

I came to the Pose Method because of injuries (damaged meniscus and cruciate ligaments, and problems with veins). After three years of heel striking, all my running injuries got worse. I couldn't move without pain and couldn't compete in a race for six months. Shifting to the new technique was for me very complicated psychologically, but the pain in my legs started to dissipate and completely disappeared after two months. I ran the Moscow Marathon in 2013 and I got a PR [personal record]—3:12 (the year before it was 3:15). Two months later, I ran the Athens Marathon. I didn't expect anything from the difficult, hilly course. I placed tenth overall with a new PR of 3:08. On top of all that, the next day I had no muscle pain or soreness.

—Yana Hmeleva, wedding planner; running experience—four years.

My philosophy emphasizing the forefoot and my critique of the modern running shoe were considered radical and clearly outside the mainstream. Then it all changed.

Let's flash forward for a little perspective and look at the current state of running. Now, the idea of nature's blueprint for running—what the Pose Method has been teaching for the last thirty-five years—has become a trend. With a proliferation of books, news stories, and magazine articles, the barrage of new rules for running has reached a tipping point, transforming the way we think about running and the shoes we choose. Some choice examples:

- The bestselling book *Born to Run,* and the stories about the Tarahumara Indians in Mexico, who run dozens of miles in simple sandals to hunt down deer.
- The work of Dr. Dan Liberman, evolutionary biologist and professor of anthropology at Harvard, whose research illustrates how the arch of the human foot evolved to provide both support and spring, making us fit for running with either minimal footwear or bare feet.
- The legendary Kenyan runners, who build stronger ankle and foot muscles and a more efficient gait by running barefoot as kids, compared with runners who grow up wearing shoes.
- Experts and top coaches making the claim that cushioned running shoes with a built-up heel make our feet lazy and our running mechanics sloppy, leading to injuries.
- Legendary track coach Vin Lananna, who used barefoot running to train his athletes, and his teams won multiple national championships at Stanford and the University of Oregon.
- The anecdotal stories about longtime runners who were plagued by injuries, then changed to minimal footwear and a forefoot landing and were cured.

These stories have not only changed the way we think about running; they've inspired people to change the way they run, transforming the marketplace. The same companies that built the wedge-heeled running shoes and promoted heel-first running mechanics are now creating minimal footwear that is nearly the opposite in design and function from the shoes they've made and sold for the last forty years. According to the *New York Times* barefoot-style shoes are now a $1.7 billion business. As the evidence keeps mounting for the new rules for running, Nike, Adidas, New Balance, and a newcomer Vibram have already made their moves to be king of the hill and successfully manage the transition.

> I was first introduced to Dr. Romanov's method after coming back from a ten-year hiatus from serious running. Prior to this break, I was continually sidelined with a laundry list of common runner's aches and pains that radiated from my feet up through the hips. My "comeback" was stalling out with the same injury issues. Dr. Romanov's method changed my running mechanics for the better through consistent drill work and practice. Within six months I was able to seamlessly incorporate these changes—such as forefoot striking rather than heel striking and pulling rather than pushing into my natural running form. Over the last five years, I have been free of injury and I am able to maintain the training required to keep me among the top competitors in the master's division of Texas.   —Jennifer Fisher

All of which is to say: For me things have come full circle. The minimalist shoes, the barefoot runners, the latest anthropological findings—all of these have aggregated to make the Pose Method I've been teaching for decades infinitely easier to share with you now.

One of my first success stories in America was in 1997. I trained Jürgen Zäck, five-time Ironman Europe winner. Jürgen explained, "I worked with Dr. Nicholas Romanov on my running form. After the session, I bent my knees a little bit. It looks like a shorter stride but it's not. My leg turnover is quicker, and my foot rests on the ground less. His new running style puts less stress on my quads and back." Jurgen improved his Ironman 26.2 miles that season from 3:03 to 2:45.

Of course, you can't just go native. Modern culture—a lifetime bound in shoes and not walking on different terrains—has caused the foot to lose some of its natural strength and functionality. So your feet—and your form—are a work in progress. For the next several weeks, you'll be learning and practicing the foundational skills you need to revolutionize your form, building up your powers of perception, strength, and balance.

Even when you hit the ground running, so to speak, you won't be clocking major mileage. If you've been running five miles a day in motion-control shoes, you may not be inclined to dial back the distance to a hundred meters a day in minimalist shoes. That's fine. After you've completed the day's lesson, feel free to put on your old shoes and run the balance of your mileage—4.5 miles, say, if the day's lesson called for a half-mile's worth of drills.

Since one of the major new skills you'll be learning is body weight perception, you can practice this skill not just when running, but also when walking, standing in line, or even sitting. This skill, as you'll learn, revolves around one simple question: Where do I feel my body weight on my feet? If you're brand-new to running, even better. Follow these lessons in order, and by the end of this book you'll be running like the best in the world.

After a disappointing Paris Marathon where an injury hampered my race, I attended a clinic with Dr. Romanov. Mastering the skills necessary for proper running technique proved to be a more time-consuming endeavor than a weekend course. Nevertheless, I persevered. Prior to working with Dr. Romanov, my marathon time was 4:04, after months of long distance training. After training with Dr. Romanov, my marathon time was 3:29, after only seven weeks of training. For me, one of the greatest benefits of learning Dr. Romanov's method is I know I will be able to enjoy a lifetime of running, where most other runners will retire after a series of injuries as they get older.

—Christine Chen

THE PERCEPTION SYSTEM

The Key to Learning

Over the next few chapters, you'll be laying the groundwork for your new running technique—refining your powers of perception, logging your observations in a journal, acquiring proper shoes, learning to film yourself running, and developing warm-up and strengthening routines. These early exercises, while easy on the cardiovascular system, are just as crucial to mastering the optimized movement patterns of the Pose Method as the running drills to come in Part Two. Each chapter—even in Part One—is designed to be approached as a training session to be revisited time and again until the concepts are fully mastered. If you're planning to keep up your running mileage as you work through these early chapters, make sure you complete your training session *before* your run, not after.

The most important element of your new running form is also the most elusive: perception. In a nutshell, perception is your ability to adapt and learn. It is an input-output system. You take in sensory information, which your brain then analyzes for decision making. When it comes to running, perception is what enables you to tune in to minor nuances in your technique. Becoming more in touch with your absolute threshold—the point where something becomes noticeable to your senses—is essential for improving your form.

A lot of runners claim they are forefoot strikers, but when they are filmed running, it is clear they are heel strikers. Their perception has not evolved enough to tell the difference between these two landings and make adjustments. To improve as a runner, you have to perceive this difference before you can make the technique adjustment on a consistent basis.

To understand the perception system you need to know how to distinguish between sense data, awareness, and feeling. At the same time, you need to know how these building blocks of perception are related and work together.

SPRINGINESS POSITION

The best way to explore these nuances of perception is to get into the basic position for all sports movements: springiness position. Your springiness position is more than just standing. It's your foundation for action, both mentally and physically.

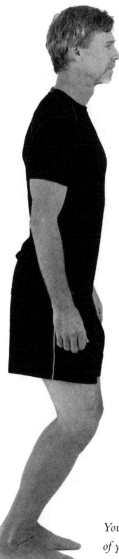

1. Take off your shoes.

2. Shift your body weight to the balls of your feet.

3. Bend your knees so they are over your toes.

4. Lean your upper body slightly forward so your shoulders are over your hips and your hips are over the balls of your feet. You can draw a direct line from the ball of the foot through the hip and shoulder joint to the ear.

5. Bend your elbows, positioning your arms above your waist, but below your shoulders.

6. Engage your core muscles, from your glutes to your shoulders, drawing your belly button toward your spine and pulling your shoulder blades together. (This is your Pose core, which will be explored in greater depth later on.)

7. Make sure that your chin is level and your eyes are looking straight ahead.

8. Mentally, give your body the cue to be ready to move, as if you were waiting for the starter's gun in a race.

Your basic athletic stance. From a wide-angle shot of your whole body, this stance communicates that you are prepared to move in any direction.

Compare your springiness position with your normal everyday stance. Do you feel more alert? More focused? More prepared to move? Excellent. You're in the ideal position to explore your powers of perception.

SENSE DATA

This aspect of perception includes all the information your senses (sight, hearing, touch, taste, smell) are capable of capturing. Maintaining springiness position, close your eyes and take note of the taste in your mouth, the brush of your clothes on your skin, and the wind or the lack of it. Keeping your weight on the balls of your feet, note how the ground feels against your skin. Open your eyes and examine what you can see directly before you. What can you smell?

Consider how your "sixth sense," proprioception, might be at work right now. While the other senses collect information from sources outside your body, your proprioception collects data from a variety of internal sources—sensory neurons located in the inner ear that signal motion and orientation of the body, receptors in the muscles, ligaments, and tendons that sustain motion and stability. Your brain is unconsciously receiving constant feedback about your movements, balance, and your body position in space. To test your proprioception, lean forward as far as you can without jutting a foot out to catch yourself. If you lose your balance resume springiness position and try again until you've internalized the limits of your balance threshold. Great athletes are in touch with proprioception like a chef is in touch with smell and taste. The more you cultivate awareness of it, the more attuned you'll be to what's happening with your body during the running process.

AWARENESS

Awareness is simply your ability to consciously register what your senses deliver. By taking note of your senses a moment ago, you engaged the awareness aspect of perception. To take it a step further, close your eyes again and listen. Can you locate the sources of the sounds you hear in relation to your body? By doing this, you are taking in sense data and using it to draw conclusions about your surroundings.

Not all sense data reaches us on a conscious level. The amount of information is too dense. When you kick a ball to someone in a soccer game, you don't think, *I'm going to move my right foot back six inches and then move it forward a half-inch off the ground to make contact, then follow through nine and a half inches.* Your sense data is being calculated into action below your thinking mind. On the other hand, most of us are not capturing all the useful sensory information that is available to our conscious mind, and like any conscious skill, the more you practice conscious awareness, the more information will become available to you. As you go through the lessons, you will focus your awareness on the key running elements.

FEELING

Feelings revolve around pleasure and pain—important feedback in training. Perceiving your feelings is what helps you distinguish between good pain and bad pain. Good pain can just mean you're having a great workout and getting the desired training effect (cardiovascular or muscular fatigue, for example). Bad pain is the acute pain of injury, meaning you should stop training and get treatment.

Returning to springiness position, take note of your feelings. Are you in pain anywhere? Is this position more or less comfortable than your everyday stance? Are you able to distinguish between the discomfort of exertion—engaging your core, in this case—and the kind of pain that needs to be remedied?

PUTTING IT ALL TOGETHER

Perception gives meaning to all the data, awareness, and feelings. It is the process that takes sense information, both conscious and unconscious, back to the brain where the raw data from the senses are gathered, analyzed, correlated, and evaluated before the body acts. Like a muscle, it needs to be trained and developed.

Great athletes are geniuses of body perception. They are deeply aware of where their body is in space and how to make adjustments to get their body from where they are to where they want to be. World-class runners have a heightened perception of how their body moves through the phases of running and how to integrate the use of their muscles in the proper sequence at the proper time. Their body is their instrument.

There is no shortcut to this process. You can read about it in a book or have coaches break down your technique, but ultimately you have to feel the nuanced changes in your body and make the adjustments. This means you have to really tune in to the running process, not zone out.

In sports and fitness, skill acquisition is connected with the development of biomechanical patterns, which is all about learning new ways to use your body. Your progress will only be as good as your perception, your ability to differentiate one movement from another. Building your runner's perception will be a part of every lesson.

Meanwhile, if you're keeping up your regular mileage in your old shoes, there's one key adjustment you can make right now: Leave your iPod at home! Tune in to the sound of your running: the sound of your feet making ground contact and the frequency of the contact. You may think that distance and time spent running are primarily physical challenges, but the fact is that runners fatigue mentally, psychologically, or spiritually before they reach a true state of physical exhaustion. The body can handle the distance, but the mind can't focus and maintain proper technique. Many of us like to use runs as a time to escape daily life, to think through problems, to get away from it all. In other words, when we run, we use our mental energy to deal with issues other than running. While this may be somewhat therapeutic, it won't make you a better runner. If your objective is to truly become a better runner, you must set aside other times to think through your life, so that you can approach your runs with a fresh and focused spirit—without tuning in to devices that enable your mind to tune out.

YOUR RUNNING JOURNAL

Tracking Your Progress

If you haven't been keeping a running journal, now's the time to start. If you have been logging your miles, now's the time to shift your focus from the quantitative measure of mileage to the qualitative evaluation of technique. Of course, everyone has their own journal personality type—that's the entire point of a journal—so whether you make your entries in a Moleskine or a composition notebook, an e-mail chain or a blog, is a decision that's entirely up to you. Whatever your favored medium, the purpose of your running journal is to set aside time to consciously focus your awareness on your running technique and the challenges and revelations of learning a new skill.

THE MIND-BODY CONNECTION

As discussed in the previous chapter on perception, your mind must be trained as rigorously as your legs. Without a signal from the mind, the first step in your running stride will not happen. And while it is possible to run at a satisfactory level by training your body and ignoring the mind, you will only reach your maximum level of performance by training your mind and your body together. Within the context of the mind's involvement in running, we can talk about three levels:

- The mental (focus and perception during your running workout)
- The psychological (lifelong behavior and attitudes you bring to running)
- The spiritual (the deep mind-body-nature connections that develop through running)

When all three are truly engaged, you will perform at your peak. Easier said than done, right?

Challenges to focus, mental discipline, and conscious control aren't just the runner's bane—they are the fundamental elements of the human condition. Deep in the psyche, the conscious and subconscious are often at odds, engaged in a kind of perpetual checks-and-balances system. This is because human beings are still animals with deeply ingrained mechanisms for survival. Your body has built-in strategies to avoid danger and protect itself from injury.

For example, on a long, hard run, the physiological, psychological, and mental fatigue associated with a maximum effort sends a danger signal to the body. What started out as a chosen and desired effort is interpreted as life threatening, something to be stopped. Your first response will not be a conscious sense of fear but rather physiological sensations. At this point, in fact, your conscious mind is still giving you full-steam-ahead signals, but the subconscious mind, intent on life preservation, begins sending the body an opposite set of instructions—muscle stiffness and pain, pounding heart, a struggle to breathe, sounds suggestive of dying. The message from the subconscious mind to the body is clear—shut it down.

In truth the situation faced by your body and colored by the subconscious mind is not life threatening. Your subconscious mind is playing it safe. But this involuntary shutdown message leaves an imprint on the conscious mind and, over time, becomes a conscious limitation. The conscious mind all too often locks in to the limited idea. That's why you always feel the same way at the four-mile mark—or wherever your limitation has become imprinted—keeping you at the same level year after year. Failure to improve is rarely a physical failure; it's almost always an entirely mental shortcoming. Then you create a reason:

- I'm just not fast.
- I'm not an elite endurance runner.
- Plateaus happen for a reason. They represent my true limit.

At every level, from the cellular on up, there is an interplay between the conscious and subconscious mind. Each has its own goals and needs. And because they seek to fulfill their own objectives through the same organism, the relations between the conscious and the subconscious are not always friendly. In order for you to improve as a runner, a truce must be declared. In order for a truce to be declared, the conscious mind must comprehend what's going on in the subconscious mind. Your running journal is the bridge and the key to peace of mind and optimal performance.

YOUR PERSONAL PROFILE

If you've been keeping a running journal, turn to the next blank page. If the spine of your new blank notebook has never been cracked, open it up now and turn to page one (or open a blank document if you're working on-screen). Under today's date, write or type in all caps: MY RUNNING LIFE—or whatever words you're comfortable looking at as the headline of your running biography. The goal of this section of your running journal is to make you consciously think about your running history and your running personality type. Approach this section the way you would a patient profile interview with your new internist. Record your best and worst experiences with the sport—your personal records, your peak mileage, your injuries and setbacks, that shoe model you loved that was discontinued five years ago, the shoe you wear now. If you're brand-new to running, say so. If you haven't run a mile since that 4:30 sprint that blew out your knee in high school, here's the place to note it. If you're comfortable writing about your fears and desires related to running, take a moment to record the peaks and valleys of those sensations throughout your running life up to now. If the prospect of journaling about emotion makes you retch, don't force yourself here—the entire point of this journal is to create a medium where you are comfortable drawing conclusions about your subconscious mind and presenting goals to bend it in the direction you need it to go. For ideas, check out the sample from a Pose Method student.

MY PERSONAL PROFILE: KURT BRUNGARDT

Even though I got to spend a lot of one-on-one time with Dr. Romanov, I had to go through my own struggles in learning Pose. I would define myself as a lifetime runner. I started running when I was in sixth grade. I did track and field in middle school and ran cross-country one year in high school, but it was just to get into shape for wrestling. Almost all wrestlers are lifetime runners.

I've run a couple of 10Ks over the years, but I didn't really train for them. I just pushed up my training mileage for a few weeks. Running is something I always liked doing. I never got the same pleasure out of biking or swimming. I liked the intense connection of my body to the earth. When I run, or more accurately jog, everything gets heightened, turned up a notch.

I've always owned a pair of running shoes, but I usually just bought the pair that was on sale. And like a good boy, I did the only thing I was ever told about running: heel strike and go from heel to toe. Running became a key piece of what I call cardio work.

I've always been a lone-wolf runner. Running was a way to escape, not a way to be social or have an affiliation. For the past twenty years, the normal running workout for me would be a thirty-minute jog. Maybe some sprint work at the end to work my max energy system and because sprinting is fun. It feels good, too, cleans out the pipes, like opening up a car on the highway to get the cobwebs out.

I've never had a running injury. I don't think this is because I have great technique. I think it's because I lift weights, jump rope, and never pushed my mileages too high. What drew me to the Pose technique was simple—since I love running, I wanted to be the best runner I could be.

If I have one overriding idea about why I want to transition to nature's way of running it is this: Heel strike is bad. Forefoot landing is good. My goal is to go from heel strike to forefoot landing. I've played around with this idea after reading books like *Born to Run* but couldn't make the shift. When I looked for books that would help me, nothing seemed to go into much detail on how to run. It was always more about how to train, not how to run. Then I met Dr. Romanov. Now I'm ready for the quest and I'm willing to go slow and be patient.

GOALS

If you have been running 400-meter repeats in seventy-five seconds, you can't just decide to run them in sixty seconds. The subconscious mind will panic and bring that ambition to a screeching halt. However, over the course of twelve to sixteen weeks, you can bring your time down a little each week, until you have made the improvement to sixty seconds—that is, if you truly believe.

Your running journal is the place to set down your long-term goals in writing so that you can then create a plan for achieving them. In addition to making the impossible possible, goals help you:

- Own the training process
- Manage your time
- Track your progress
- Make adjustments when results don't meet expectations

As you move through the program, you'll be setting both long-term and short-term goals that are realistic, measurable, and have specific completion dates. Inevitably, some will have to be revised, and the act of tweaking plans and expectations will further refine the powers of perception so crucial to your success as a runner.

For today's journal entry, under the heading GOALS, I simply want you to describe what impelled you to pick up this book and embark on the Pose Method program. What do you hope to attain in the next ten weeks? Ten months? Ten years? Whether your goals are as broad as a lifetime of injury-free running or as specific as a sub-three-hour marathon, now is the time to put it in writing.

GOALS

My goal is to learn these new rules for running. It's accepted now that heel striking and overstriding are the cause of so many running injuries and inefficiencies. My goal is to clear out these bad habits and run with precise and perfect technique. I don't clock mileage, so it's all about improving technique to me. I want to hit that zone where running feels effortless, like I'm being run instead of running, not to get too Zen.

When you get to Part Two, you'll have the opportunity to come up with a detailed training schedule that will carry you through the Pose Method program and beyond. The long-term goals you write here will help you gauge the intensity and scope of your short-term goals down the line.

FOCUS PREPARATION

Your running journal is a great tool for narrowing your focus in preparation for a training session. Here is where you can put down in words what you want to focus on in your upcoming session. For today's entry, choose one aspect of the last chapter's perception exercise that you'd like to repeat—your balance threshold, for example. Under the FOCUS PREPARATION heading, list the steps you plan to take to improve your proprioception awareness, what sensations you expect to associate with the limits of your balance threshold.

FOCUS PREPARATION

My goal is keep it simple, stupid. I've struggled with distinguishing the simplest thing: Am I landing on my heel or forefoot first? This makes me feel very incompetent. So today I'm going to get into my springiness position and just shift my weight back and forth between my heels and my forefoot and try to really zero in on the difference. First I will do large shifts that are simple to feel with a longish gap of time between shifts, like maybe two seconds. Then make the shifts more subtle and faster.

Now put this book and your journal down and carry out the exercise.

POST-SESSION REVIEW

This is where you break down your lessons and your runs—what you did right and what you did wrong, epiphanies you had, and struggles you contended with. Don't shy away from regular journal stuff, too, like how far you ran, your course, your time, what you ate, and how your body feels.

For today's purposes, I want you to reflect on the perception exercise you just revisited. How did it feel this time around as opposed to last time? Were you focused, or did your mind seem to wander? Did you feel any pain or other discomfort? Write all your observations down under the heading POST-SESSION THOUGHTS.

POST-SESSION THOUGHTS

So, this was easy. I stayed focused and attuned to the shift of my weight from heel to forefoot and back. But then again, I wasn't moving my feet. Honestly, I felt a little bored. I need to remember my promise to myself: Be patient. And always be grateful if I gain an insight, even if I struggle holding on to it. What I want to do is keep this same focus when I start moving. I want to carry this focus into jogging.

Writing about an activity you've just completed has value far beyond the document it provides about your progress. This is the aspect of journal keeping that cultivates mindfulness and focus on the present moment—a crucial skill when it comes to pushing your body beyond perceived limits.

While it's nice to think that you can put your body on autopilot and run beautifully while your mind goes on vacation, things rarely work that way. The most common flight the mind takes during a long run is toward the future. The body may be at mile six of a marathon, but the mind begins to calculate what might happen at mile eighteen. Instead of monitoring the present performance of the body, the mind starts a whole system of conjectures about how ready the body might be to get through the whole marathon in good shape.

By thinking ahead of the present position, the mind is building up a substantial fear of the future, while the physiological and biomechanical processes of the body, untended by the conscious mind here at mile six, begin to break down because of the lack of attention.

When the mind returns to the present from its visit to the future, it finds a physical process in disarray, creating something of a self-fulfilling prophecy. First the mind was concerned about the body's ability to get all the way to the finish line in good form, and then it returns to the present to find things already falling apart long before the finish line.

At this point, it is usually too late to rescue a good performance. After all, the signals now coming to the brain from the body are distress signals: The stride has broken down, muscles are sore, et cetera. The mind, which already had developed a fear of the future, now has those fears confirmed, all because it left the present realm and went off on its own to explore the future.

Now imagine what happens for the runner who logs this experience in a journal immediately afterward. The conscious movement from the present to the future and back to the present is noted. *Things began to fall apart at mile six, not long after the worry about mile eighteen took hold.* By mapping out the sequence of thoughts and sensations in narrative form, your mind takes back ownership of the very situation that got out of its control. You'll note these mental pratfalls as things to avoid in your Focus Preparation entry the next time you prepare to run. And during your next run, you'll be less inclined to let your mind wander off into the same places that got you in trouble the last time around.

REFRAME

Reframing turns a potential negative situation into a positive takeaway. It functions under the premise that it's not about what happened; it's about how you think about what happened. Let's say you just had a bad run and you feel discouraged. You have to reframe the situation by asking yourself these questions:

- What did I do well?
- What did I learn?
- What can I use that I learned?

You just have to find one positive thing. It could even be that you did your workout instead of surfing the Internet. Finding and documenting the positive keeps you coming back.

REFRAME

Today, I showed up and did the exercise, even though there was a voice in my head that said I don't need to do this simple exercise. I got it out of my head and let my body experience. I won't let my mind trick me; this is all about embodiment, getting out of my head and into my body.

THOUGHTS AND FEELINGS

This is a free-form heading under which you can reflect on running and the Pose Method. Here is where you write down the running revelation you have at three a.m. and don't want to forget. Maybe you'll take it deeper by writing about it more the next day. This could also be your personal comments page where you respond to something you read or heard about running technique. Or something you see out on the course that you find annoying or inspiring.

THOUGHTS AND FEELINGS

Oh my God, I was walking downstairs today at work and all of a sudden I became aware of how I was landing on the ball of my foot with each step and this made going down the stairs easy. Then I realized that for every activity there must be an optimal way for applying my body weight. I can apply this to so many things in life and sports.

The rest of this book is filled with directions about what you should be recording in your journal and how you should be framing your approach to the Pose Method, but this section belongs entirely to you and your free-flowing consciousness. Let it wander here so that it doesn't wander when you're running or reflecting on your form.

CHOOSING AND USING THE RIGHT SHOE . . . OR NONE AT ALL

Finding the Perfect Fit

Now that you've been introduced to the powers of perception and documentation, the following statement probably sounds painfully obvious: If you wear heavily cushioned shoes with thick, inflexible soles, you will not be able to run according to nature's blueprint and your chances of injury will increase. Motion-control shoes disable your foot's natural abilities and muscle activity, keeping it rigid, instead of allowing the foot to move freely. Constrained feet are weak feet. They are not a runner's friend. So how is it that the athletic shoe has played such a powerful role in American sports and culture over the last forty years? The shoe you choose to put on your foot has become a partner in a deep and existential relationship, a statement about identity, status, even politics. Runners are no exception: We feel a deep conviction that the shoes we wear are our ticket to improved performance. This has more to do with marketing than reality.

Exploiting our sneaker worship tendencies, the major running-shoe companies have been engaged in a decades-long technology war over the latest and greatest in alleged performance-enhancing features—whatever new type of heel (gels, springs, air bubbles) and construction (arch support, motion control) deemed necessary to stay ahead of the curve. These shoes feel comfy on your feet, just like comfort food tastes good. But all the padding, stiff support, and motion control make them like a cast, something you would wear if you were injured, but not a smart choice for a healthy foot. In fact, this design will turn a healthy foot into a weak, poorly functioning foot. They even have top-secret labs where new gimmicks are developed and market tested for optimum revenue increase, regardless of what is truly good for the runner.

Fortunately, the latest and greatest is now all about simplicity. Now you can easily get your hands on the pair of flat running shoes you'll need to learn the Pose Method.

But before you throw out your gel-filled, high-stability, five-pound shoes, put them on and pull out your running journal. Under the RUNNER PROFILE heading, describe how these running shoes feel on your feet. How is your mobility with the shoes on as compared with your mobility barefoot? When you press your feet against the ground, can you feel the points of contact, or is the pressure uniform across the soles of your feet? Take these notes with you when you go to purchase the type of running shoe endorsed by me and this book.

THE RIGHT RUNNING SHOE: FLAT, THIN, AND FLEXIBLE

To maximize performance and minimize injury, you want to buy a light shoe with a sole that is flat, thin, and flexible. This allows you to develop a very precise, refined interaction between your foot and the ground—an impossible feat with a thick and inflexible shoe sole. In a movement where every hundredth of a second counts, neuromuscular coordination is crucial for getting on and off support quickly. Excess cushioning delays this process, and as a consequence, running technique deteriorates.

Visit the running shoe section of any sports store these days, and you will encounter a confounding array of options—very few (if any) of which involve the words "flat," "thin," or "flexible." To obtain a flat shoe, you'll need to ask for a zero-millimeter heel lift or toe drop. For a thin, flexible shoe, you'll need to select a model from the barefoot or minimalist category.

Always lace running shoes tight from the arch up to the ankle, leaving the laces looser at the toes and balls of your feet. The fit should be snug—not so tight that your toes are crunched, but not so loose that they're wiggling around in space, either.

Once you've found a pair that seems right, put them to the test with the perception exercise you learned in the previous chapter. Trust me—the sales clerk has seen everything under the sun and won't bat an eye if you assume springiness position and close your eyes a few times. Next, jog in place and see if you can feel each landing. Which part of your foot is first making contact—heel, midfoot, or forefoot? Where do you feel your weight when you land—in front of your body, beneath your body, or behind your body? Are your shoulders rounded or pulled back toward your spine? What's your head position? If the shoes you're trying on bother you in any way as you contemplate these questions—or if they dull your senses in a manner similar to your old running shoes—take them off and ask for another model.

On the other hand, if it feels like kismet between you and the shoe, try jogging a few strides on the balls of your feet. You should find that the entire shoe bends with your foot—no rubbing from the shoelaces, no resistance in the bend of the soles.

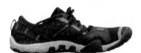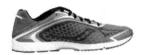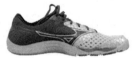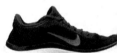

Some flat minimalist shoe models to consider

BAREFOOT RUNNING

If you study the running form of successful African runners who have dominated the world's distance scene for much of the past four decades, you'll see that their movements are a model of efficiency and grace. In most cases, this form resulted from barefoot running as a child, which led to developing proper running technique and strength around the ankles and feet. Developing this strength, instead of buying it in the form of a shoe, will greatly reduce your chances of being sidelined by Achilles tendonitis, plantar fasciitis, or other common runners' injuries. However, you should think of barefoot running as a training tool, not a miracle. Taking off your shoes or donning a pair of snug five-fingered running socks will increase your proprioception and sensitivity to your running gait but it won't guarantee proper technique. It is possible to complete many of this book's lessons barefoot, and I encourage you to do so whenever the mood strikes—particularly for the jumping and jump rope drills, or whenever you have a beach, a track, or a golf course handy. But I must stress that a barefoot runner does not a Pose runner make. You'll need the Pose Method for that.

ORTHOTICS: HOW TO DITCH 'EM?

When you break your leg, do you stay in a cast for life? The obvious answer is no. The same goes for wearing orthotics.

In theory orthotics are designed to correct abnormalities, such as flat feet or high arches, and to treat iliotibial band syndrome and knee pain. In reality they are an artificial solution that treats a symptom and doesn't cure the real cause. Orthotics miss the main issues: developing your weak body link and improving your running technique. Instead, they allow already weak muscles to deteriorate, and they decrease your ability to perceive proper technique corrections. Choosing orthotics is choosing to use a crutch for life.

Still, it's one thing to know that orthotics are not helpful and it's another thing to stop wearing them after many years of relying on the support they provide. Getting rid of your orthotics can be challenging. You need to do it gradually and safely. Here are some guiding principles:

- First of all, try to reduce your fear. Remind yourself that your orthotics haven't been solving the problem; they've been masking it.
- Complete the remaining exercises in Part One with your orthotics inserted in your new minimalist shoes.
- Starting with Part Two—the lessons—remove your orthotics. If you feel pain, put them back in your shoes and try removing them during the next lesson.
- Go slow, you need to retrain your feet, making them strong, flexible, and responsive.
- During this transition period train at low mileages.

Selected History of Running Shoes

Straw & Leather

BC — Early footwear seen as far back as 7000 BC, 3000 BC, and around 300 BC on the Greeks and Romans

1852 — The first known leather shoes to have spikes

Vulcanized Rubber & Spikes

1916 — Keds athletic shoes are released, the first mainstream sneakers

1917 — First Converse All-Stars

1936 — Adidas produces the spiked running shoe worn by Jesse Owens in the Berlin Olympics

Wedge Midsole & Traction

1972 — Bill Bowerman uses first Nike shoe with the Oregon Track Team

1975 — Bill Bowerman and Nike introduce 'jogging' to the US market with the wedge midsole running shoe

Cushioning: Air, Gels, & Springs

1980s — Nike releases the Nike Air with increased cushion under the heel

 1990s — Gel inserts are introduced as a way to increase comfort & support

2000s — Springed shoes are the next step in added impact support

Minimalist Footwear Returns

 2008 — Shoes with minimal support return to the market, focusing on a more natural approach

2010 — Zero Drop shoes are released with a flat design across the bottom

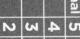

DIGITAL CAPTURE

Getting to Know Your Stride

Now that you know how important perception is to a runner and how a well-kept running journal and the right footwear will optimize your perception, I want to teach you about one of the best tools for testing those perception skills: filming yourself. Once limited to the highest echelons of coaching and team sports, game film can now be generated for anyone in possession of a smartphone and an able-bodied friend.

Like the classic before-and-after advertising campaign, your running films will give you a clear sense of your progress, as well as an indication of what areas you'll need to focus on most in order to keep improving. To attain this, you'll first need to record your baseline. Everybody has to start somewhere, and it's always a good idea to document where that is before you reform your ways.

BASIC FILMING PROCEDURE

In an ideal world you would have a video camera and a tripod for shooting, but your smartphone is fine. You don't have to recruit a future Spielberg to wield it—a friend will do nicely. If you have kids, they're already Spielbergs, so grab one of them.

Next, scout out a location that you can return to again and again throughout your journey into the Pose Method. This will enable you to have clearer points of comparison when it comes time to review multiple film sessions. The location should be relatively flat and wide open so that your cameraperson can stand in one place and train the lens on you without obstruction for at least twenty meters. An added bonus would be if the running surface were suitable for running barefoot. If you have a track or a sandy stretch of beach nearby, use it.

Lastly, wear an outfit that will contrast with the background of the place you are running, so your feet, legs, and joints stand out in the video.

Once you've got your camera operator, your location, and your clothes picked out, throw on your new running shoes and start the camera rolling.

1. Use a couple of white T-shirts or other highly visible objects to mark the beginning and end of the video capture segment. These should be spaced twenty to forty meters apart.

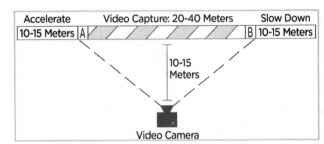

Video capture setup: give yourself 10–15 meters to accelerate to moderate speed before you enter the camera's frame.

2. Stand at the halfway point between these two objects. The camera should be positioned so your entire body, from head to toe, can be seen in the frame.

3. The camera should then be trained on the first marker ("A" in the illustration).

4. Give yourself ten to fifteen meters to get up to a moderate speed—the pace you would hold if you were running a half marathon—before you reach the first marker and enter the camera's frame.

5. Once you're in the frame, the cameraperson, staying in the same spot, pans to follow you for twenty to forty meters, keeping you centered in the frame without zooming in at any point.

6. As you pass the second marker ("B" in the illustration) the cameraperson should stop panning, allowing you to run out of the frame of the camera.

7. You should continue running for ten to twenty more meters.

8. Repeat the sequence at a much faster pace—not an all-out sprint, but around your 5K race speed.

If you have the time, you can expand your running footage by completing the same sequence barefoot. For more extensive analysis, have your camera operator film you from front and back as well.

If you can't snag a camera operator but can get your hands on a tripod, place the tripod assembly far enough back so that markers "A" and "B" are both in the frame. Begin recording, and then run the sequence as directed above.

CREATING A SCHEDULE FOR FILMING

As a general rule, you should film yourself anytime you feel like you need feedback about your form. At the very least, you should plan on recording on these occasions:

- Today, to establish your baseline form
- In the workout phase of Lesson One and after you've completed Lesson Ten
- At the end of each three-week segment of the running circuit as you build up the mileage and hone your form

If you have a tripod, you might also consider filming yourself every week, practicing the drills that accrue throughout the lessons. Increase the frequency to the beginning and end of every week throughout the program, and you'll have an incredible wealth of footage to study and improve on.

Being able to step outside yourself and analyze your technique will help you quickly see the difference between what you think you're doing and what you're really doing. Before you know it, you'll be analyzing how *everyone* is running. Your friends may give you a quizzical look when you point out a nice forefoot strike, but landing on your forefoot and being able to analyze it will improve your running. There is no better way to discover whether you're aligning with or deviating from the standard perfect running form.

SIX-POINT RUNNING ANALYSIS

The graphic on page 204 is a handy visual reference for analyzing your running form. Analyzing film, like running, is a skill; the more you do it the better you'll get at it. This graphic will cover the basics. This topic will be covered in more detail in the chapter called Becoming Your Own Coach.

PREPARE TO MOVE

Increasing Your Mobility

According to an ancient Chinese saying, "You are as old as your joints." If your joints have a full range of motion and move without pain, your movement has the quality of youth.

To attain this, your joints, muscles, and tendons need to be strong enough to absorb, load, and release energy back into movement. The routine in this chapter will build a foundation for increasing your joint mobility and improving muscle-tendon elasticity—essential qualities for preventing injuries and improving performance.

The dynamic movements you are about to learn are a little different from the conventional stretching methods you were taught in high school—methods based on the antiquated notion that muscles can be stretched and lengthened. From anatomy textbooks it is well-known that a muscle's length is fixed and determined by the size of the supporting bones and joints. Flexibility, by the meaning of the two words—"flex" and "ability"—is the ability to freely move the joints. The key to flexibility, as it relates to muscles, is their ability to relax, allowing your joints to move. In this respect, I am appealing not to muscles, but to joints. The muscles support and empower joint movement. This type of mobility work requires a different mind-set than traditional stretching. Gentle stretching with short holds can also relax the muscle involved, releasing tension, which in turn makes the muscle not *longer,* per se, but more *responsive.* By freeing up the movement potential of your joints, you will improve your functional mobility, allowing you to move through larger ranges of motion. This has nothing to do with stretching your muscles.

As you progress through the movement preparation routine, it's important to keep one rule in mind: You want to place the bulk of your body weight on the area that is *not* being moved or worked. For example, if you're working on your right ankle, you want all your body weight on your left foot for support. Eventually, once you've gained mobility in your right ankle, you can shift some weight to that ankle and move it through its range of motion with a load (your body weight). Like a progressive resistance program, you can add more body weight to the area you're working as the joint, tendons, and muscles become stronger. But never sacrifice range of motion or safety. Add more weight just a little at a time, over a period of weeks or even months. The first priority here is to increase your mobility.

As with any new program, the moves may feel awkward at first. Because the photos illustrate the most advanced versions of these positions, you're not likely to mirror them exactly from the start. Take heart: Your range of motion will increase through consistent effort. Meanwhile, try to channel any uneasiness into your on-going efforts to improve perception—perception of your body weight and where it can be most effectively applied, and perception of your range of motion.

Here are some movement preparation guidelines:

• You'll complete this routine before every lesson and every workout.
• You are performing the action of bending at your joints.
• The entire routine should take eight to ten minutes to complete.
• As you become comfortable with this routine, try letting one move flow into the next, so the individual stretches become one nonstop motion.

HAND STRETCH/WRIST EXTENSION

1. Position your right arm as if carrying a large serving tray—elbow bent, palm up, fingers pointed forward.

2. Use your left hand to pull your fingers down, unbending your right arm until it is fully extended before you and your fingers are being pulled back toward your body. Think of lengthening and pulling simultaneously.

3. Repeat with the other hand.

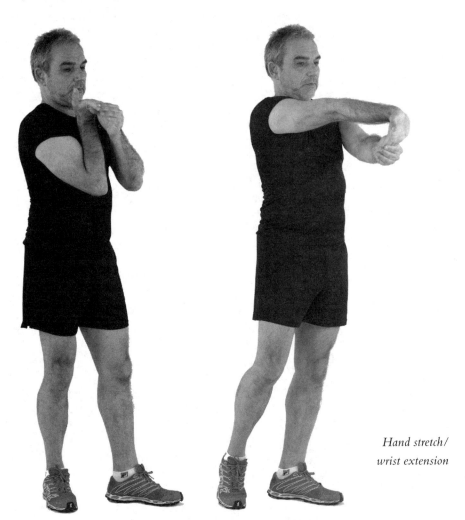

Hand stretch/ wrist extension

HAND STRETCH/WRIST EXTENSION ELBOWS IN

1. Interlace your fingers in front of your chest, palms turned down, elbows pointing outward.

2. Rotate your palms up, keeping your shoulders down as you bring your elbows together. Don't worry if you can't make your elbows touch together. Be patient; your range of motion will improve with time.

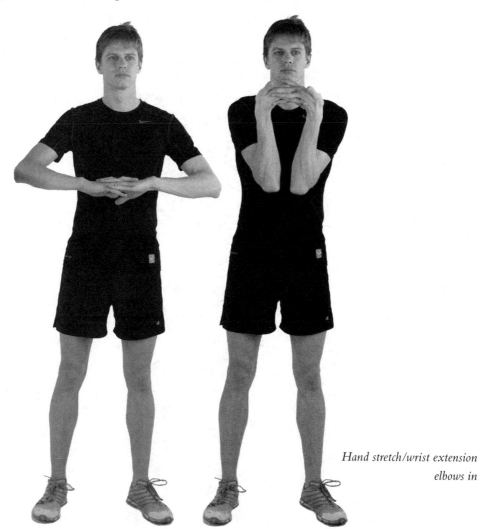

*Hand stretch/wrist extension
elbows in*

HAND AND ARM STRETCH/ WRIST EXTENSION OUTWARD

1. Interlace your fingers, palms facing outward.

2. Straighten your arms in front of your chest at shoulder level. Keeping your shoulder blades back and down, feel the movement in your shoulders, elbows, wrists, and hands. Don't round your back.

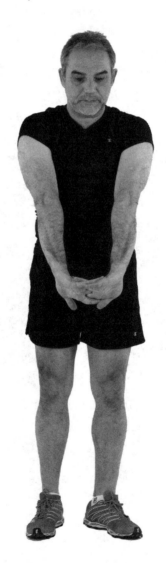

Hand and arm stretch/wrist extension outward

WRIST MOBILITY: PRAYER POSITION

1. With hands in prayer position, place arms in front of chest, elbows pointing outward with hands touching chest.

2. Press your fingertips against each other with equal pressure. The bottoms of your palms will slightly separate and your elbows will gently rise a few inches. Feel the pressure on each individual fingertip, keeping your shoulders down and relaxed.

Wrist mobility: prayer position

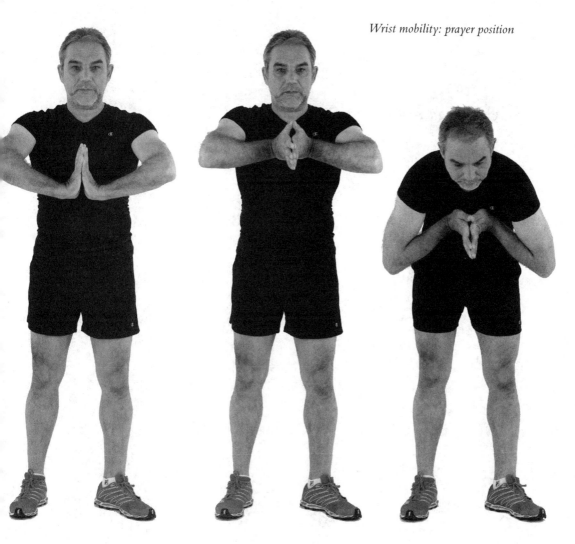

INTERLACED WRIST ROTATION

1. With your arms extended in front of you, cross your hands, bringing your left hand over your right, palms facing, and interlace your fingers. Keep shoulders level and don't round your back.

2. Rotate hands in toward your chest and then back out in full extension.

3. Repeat, crossing right hand over left.

Interlaced wrist rotation

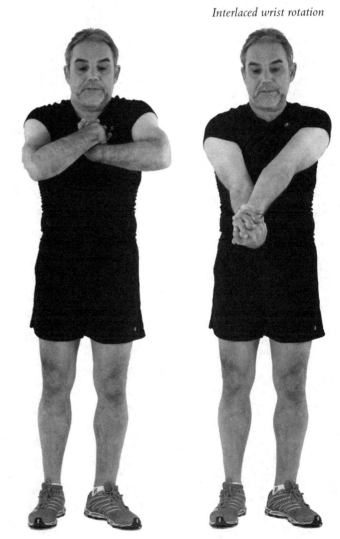

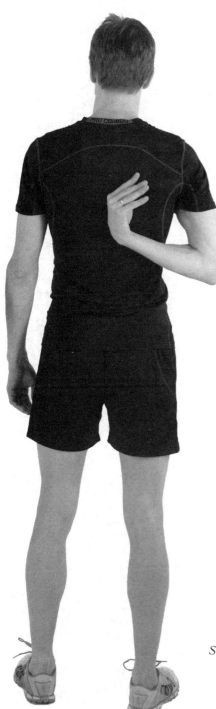

SHOULDER BLADE TOUCH

1. Place one hand behind your back, as if you're about to scratch it.

2. Keeping your shoulders down and relaxed, reach your hand to touch the shoulder blade. Don't bend at the waist.

3. Repeat with the other hand. Note that it's common for one side to be easier than the other.

Shoulder blade touch

DOUBLE SHOULDER BLADE TOUCH

1. Place both hands behind your back.

2. Keeping your shoulders down and relaxed and taking care not to bend at the waist, touch your shoulder blades. (Right hand touches right shoulder blade, left hand touches left shoulder blade.) Again, it's common for one side to be easier than the other.

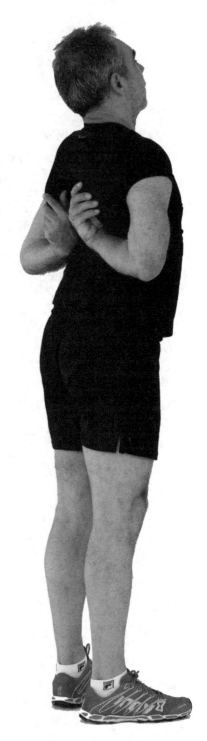

Double shoulder blade touch

REACH AND GRAB

1. Place your left hand behind your back. Place your right hand behind your back by reaching over right shoulder.

2. Without rounding or arching your back, bring hands toward each other, allowing your fingers to lock. If your hands can't lock in a grip, bring them as close to touching as you can.

3. Switch hands and repeat.

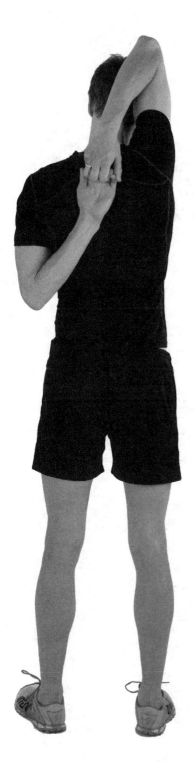

Reach and grab

REVERSE PRAYER

1. Place both arms behind your back.

2. Bring palms together, fingers up, into prayer position, careful to avoid rounding or arching your back or bending at the waist. If your hands can't achieve prayer position, bring your palms as close together as you can. Again, be patient. This move requires a lot of mobility in your shoulder joints.

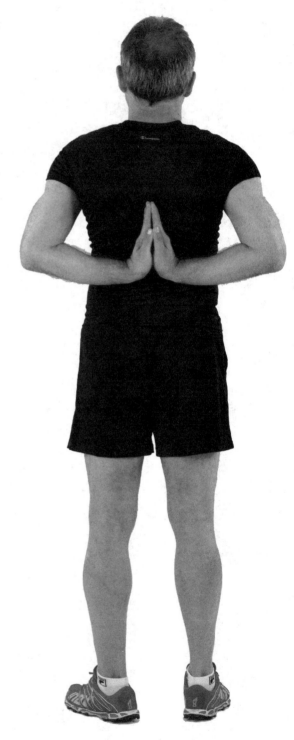

Reverse prayer

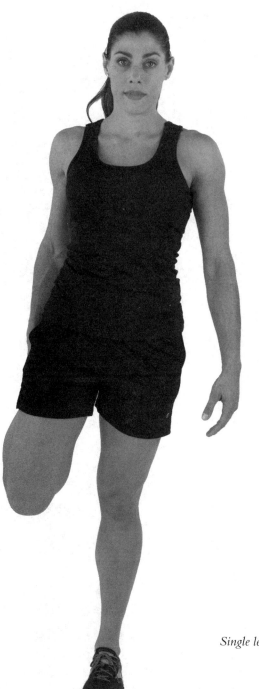

SINGLE LEG QUAD MOBILITY

1. Stand with your feet shoulder-width apart.

2. Balancing on your right leg, reach back and grab your left foot (just below the ankle) with your left hand. On your right leg—your support leg—keep your ankle, hip, shoulder, and ear aligned. Don't arch your back. Keep your thighs lined up next to each other and your left leg in line with the hip.

3. Pull your left foot toward your left buttock. Be gentle; don't force your heel to touch your buttock. Range of motion will improve with time.

4. Repeat with the other leg.

Single leg quad mobility

SINGLE LEG QUAD MOBILITY WITH FLOOR TOUCH

1. Balance on your right leg, holding your left leg behind you (same as the starting position in the previous exercise). Again, don't force your heel to touch your buttock.

2. Bend forward gently, letting your right arm—your free arm—swing forward ahead of your shoulder. Feeling your support leg rooted to the ground for balance, look toward the ground as you bend further until you're able to touch the ground with your right hand—your free hand—aiming for a spot a few inches in front of your toes.

3. Switch legs and repeat.

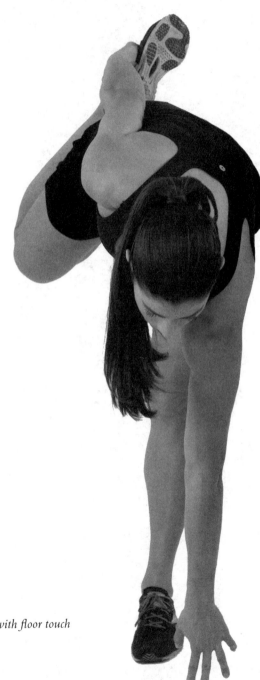

Single leg quad mobility with floor touch

DEEP FRONT LUNGE

1. Stand with your feet shoulder-width apart.

2. Step forward with your right leg. The heel of your back foot should be off the ground.

3. Lower your hips (your center of gravity) toward the ground, ideally creating a 90-degree angle with your knee joint. Be patient if you can't make 90 degrees. Your range of motion will improve with time.

4. Repeat with your left leg.

Deep front lunge

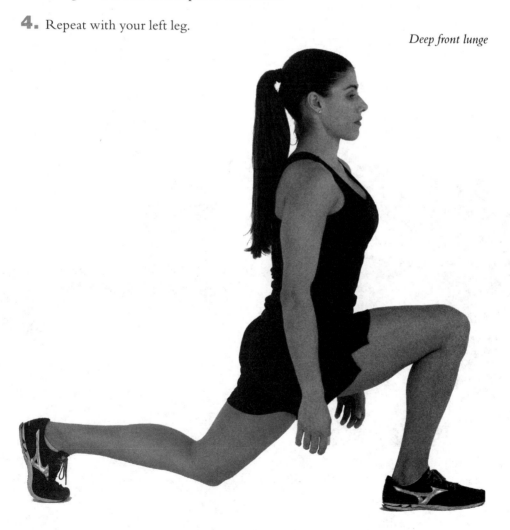

THE SPIDERMAN

1. Stand with hands on hips, then step forward with your right leg. The heel of your back foot should be off the ground (same as deep front lunge position).

2. From this position, bend forward, bringing your arms inside your front leg, attempting to touch the ground with both forearms and elbows. You'll probably need to work up to this range of motion. In the beginning, as you bring your arms inside your legs, you may have to put one or both hands on the ground for support before you can drop down to both elbows.

3. Repeat with your left leg.

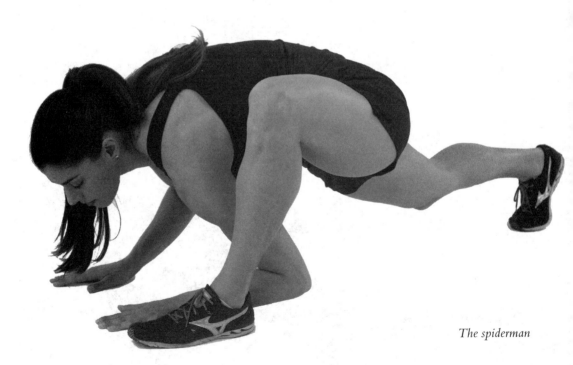

The spiderman

SIDE TO SIDE SQUAT WITH ARM OUT

1. From a standing position, bend forward at the waist, putting both hands on the ground in front of you for support, and sit back into a squatting position.

2. Reach your arms out in front of you, clasping your fingers together.

3. Shift your weight onto your left leg as you extend your right leg out to the side. On your extended leg, your foot points straight up and your body weight is on your heel. Try to make your movements from side to side precise and fluid, feeling the movement deep in your hips.

4. Repeat with the other leg.

Side to side squat with arm out

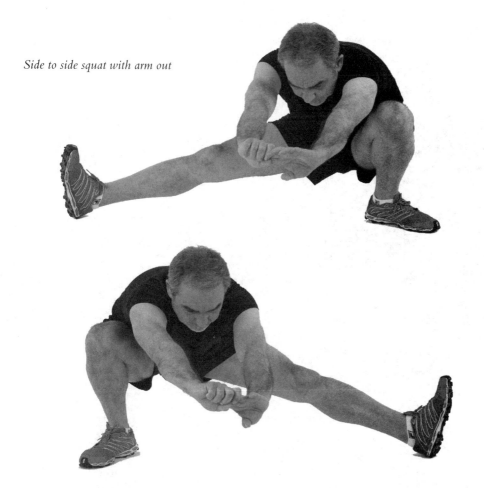

SIDE SQUAT WITH FLOOR REACH

1. Start from the sideways deep squat stretch position from the above exercise with your right leg extended to the side.

2. Now bend forward, letting your head drop down as you extend your arms straight out and rest your palms on the ground.

4. To increase the stretch, inch your fingers forward.

5. Repeat with the other leg extended.

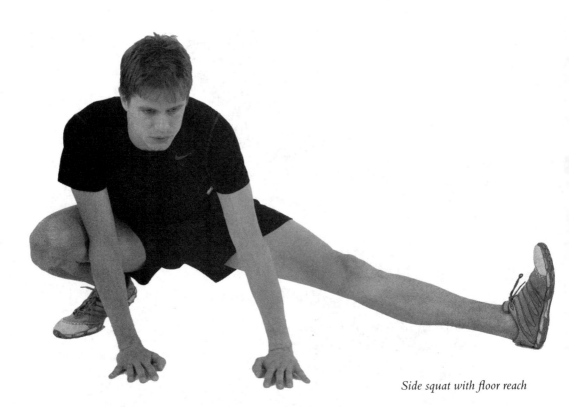

Side squat with floor reach

SIDE SQUAT WITH TOE TOUCH

1. Start from the sideways deep squat stretch position with your right leg extended.

2. Rotate your chest toward your left knee as you reach your right arm toward your extended foot.

3. Extend your left arm beyond the inside of your left knee, making sure you breathe as you hold this position. Your left hand may touch the ground for support if you need it.

4. Repeat with the other leg extended.

Side squat with toe touch

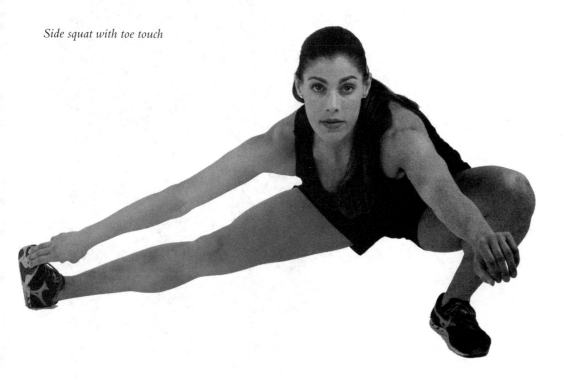

FLOOR TOUCH: ONE FOOT BACK

1. Stand with feet shoulder–width apart. Step forward with your right foot, bringing it about six inches in front of your left foot.

2. Bend forward, touching the ground with your hands.

3. Repeat with the other foot.

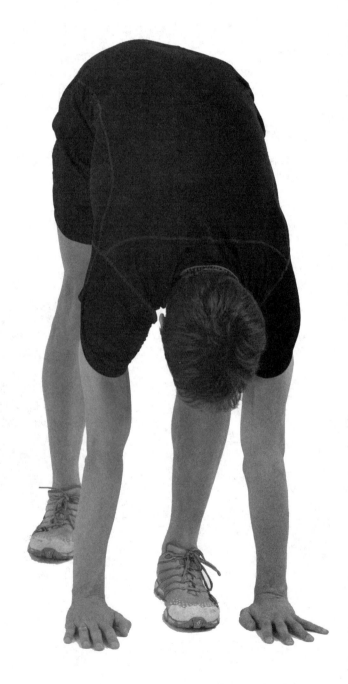

Floor touch: one foot back

FLOOR TOUCH: TOE TO HEEL INLINE

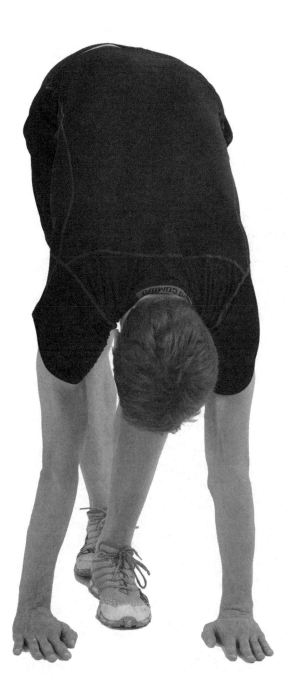

1. Stand with one foot directly in front of the other, heel of the front foot touching the toe of the back foot.

2. Bend forward, touching the ground with your hands.

3. Repeat with the front foot and the back foot reversed.

Floor touch: toe to heel inline

FLOOR TOUCH: ONE FOOT FORWARD TOES UP

1. Stand with feet shoulder–width apart. Step forward with your right foot, bringing it about six inches in front of your left foot. Toes of your front foot should be raised up, weight equally distributed on both feet.

2. Bend forward, touching the ground with your hands.

3. Repeat with the other foot.

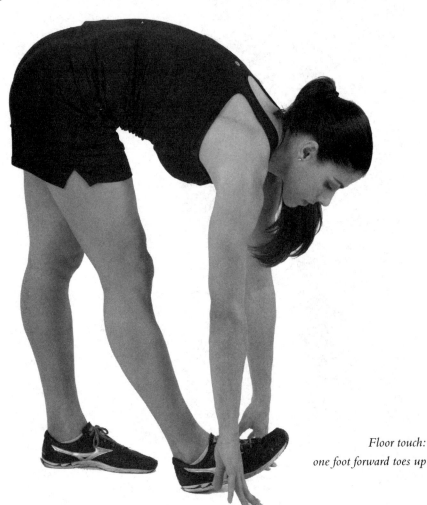

Floor touch:
one foot forward toes up

FLOOR TOUCH: DUAL SUPINATION TOES UP

1. Stand with feet together (parallel), toes raised, weight on heels.

2. Bend forward, touching the ground with your hands.

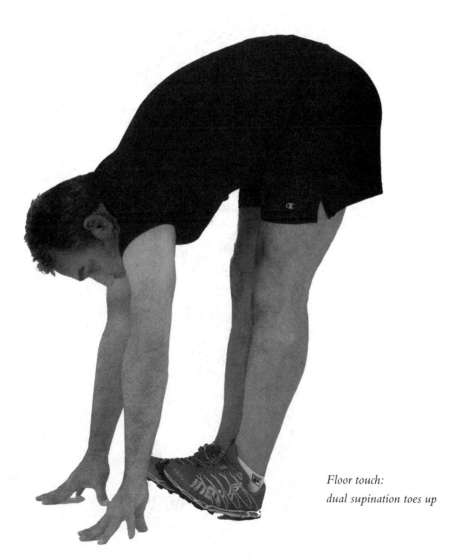

Floor touch:
dual supination toes up

FLOOR TOUCH: ANKLE CROSS

1. Stand with your right leg crossed over your left, feet side by side, flat on the ground.

2. Bend forward, touching the ground with your hands.

3. Repeat with the other leg crossed.

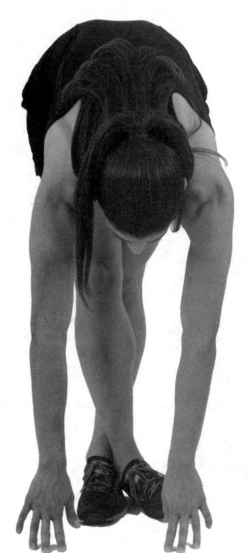

Floor touch: ankle cross

FLOOR TOUCH: ANKLE CROSS DUAL SUPINATION

1. Stand with your right leg crossed over your left, feet raised up along their outside edges (lateral side).

2. Bend forward, touching the ground with your hands.

3. Repeat with the other leg crossed.

Floor touch:
ankle cross dual supination

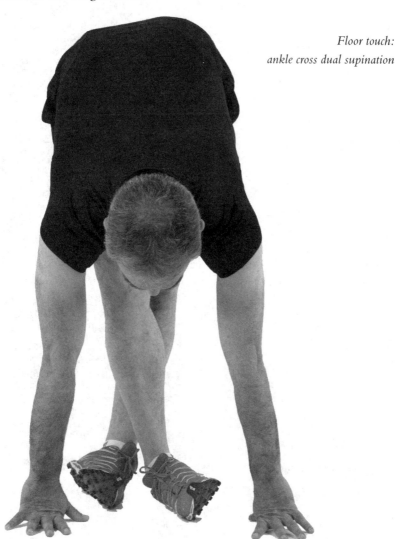

FLOOR TOUCH: ONE FOOT FORWARD SUPINATION

1. Stand with feet shoulder-width apart. Step forward with your right foot, bringing it about six inches in front of your left foot. Tilt the front foot onto its outside edge.

2. Bend forward, touching the ground with your hands.

3. Repeat with the other foot.

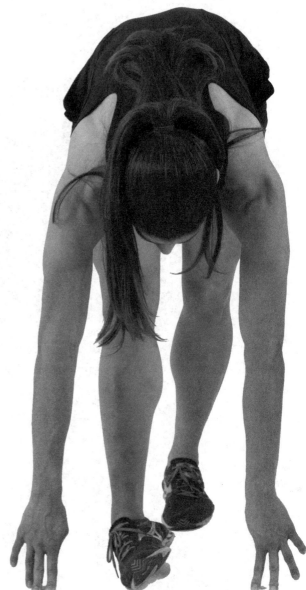

Floor touch: one foot forward supination

FLOOR TOUCH: DUAL SUPINATION

1. Stand with feet together (parallel), both feet tilted onto their outside edges.

2. Bend forward, touching the ground with your hands.

Floor touch: dual supination

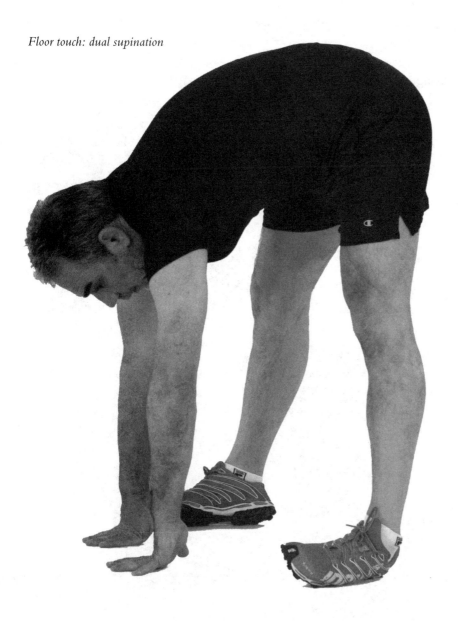

STANDING FORWARD BEND: HANDS CLASPED UP

1. Stand with feet together and flat on the floor, hands behind your back with fingers interlaced. Let your arms naturally hang down (your hands will be close to your tailbone).

2. Bend forward, bringing your forehead toward your knees as your arms rise and naturally follow the bending movement.

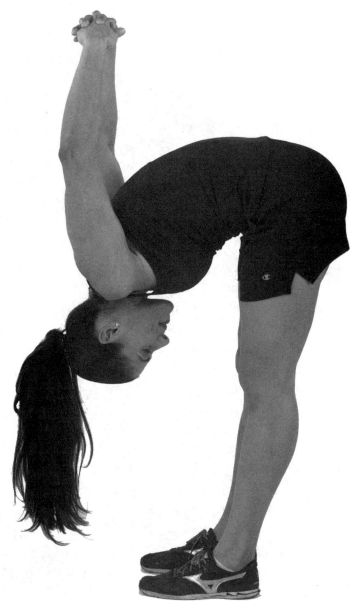

Standing forward bend: hands clasped up

FLOOR TOUCH: FEET OUT

1. Stand with heels together, feet flat, toes pointing out (first position in ballet). Hands should be hanging at your sides.

2. Bend forward, touching the ground with your hands.

Floor touch: feet out

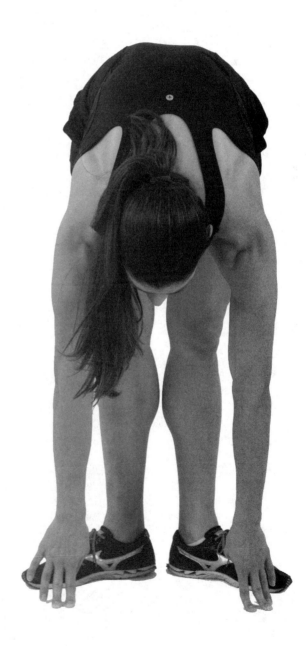

FLOOR TOUCH: FEET OUT
ANKLE CROSS

1. Place your right foot in front of your left foot, so that the heel of your right foot is near the arch of your back (left) foot (same as third position in ballet). Arms hang at your sides.

2. Bend forward at the waist, touching the ground with your hands.

3. Repeat with the other foot in front.

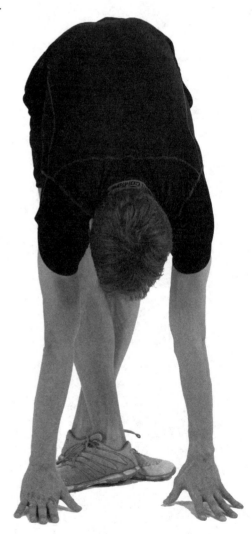

Floor touch:
feet out ankle cross

STANDING FORWARD BEND:
ANKLE TOUCH

1. Stand with feet wide apart, hands at your sides.

2. Bend forward, grabbing your ankles and moving your head toward the floor just in front of your toes.

Standing forward bend:
ankle touch

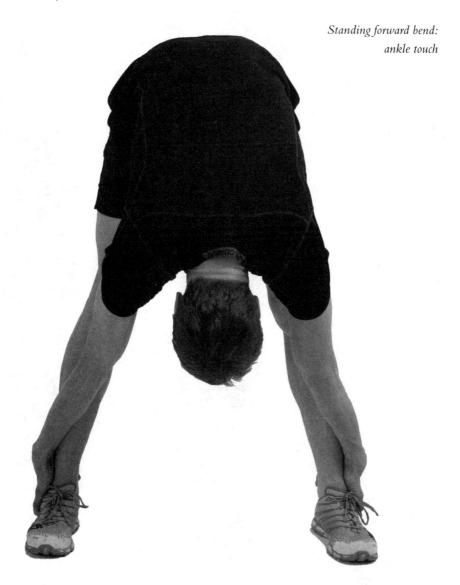

BASE JUMP IN PLACE

1. Start in your springiness position—standing with your weight on the balls of your feet, knees over toes, ankles, hips, shoulders, and ears all in alignment.

2. Jump straight up, raising your shoulders slightly to aid liftoff, maintaining springiness position as your feet leave the ground. Think of this as an *unweighting* motion rather than a jump.

3. Land on the balls of your feet, staying off heels.

4. Repeat for a set of eight, keeping ground contact short and your upper body relaxed.

5. Rest for one minute.

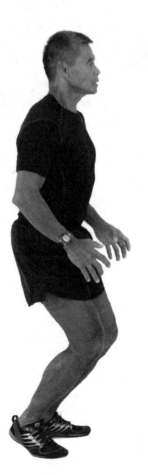

*Base jump in place.
Shoulder shrug aids the
unweighting sequence.*

HEEL TOUCH JUMP

1. Start in your springiness position, then drop your arms so they hang loosely at your sides.

2. Jump straight up, raising your shoulders slightly to aid liftoff, maintaining springiness position throughout the movement.

3. Touch your heels together at the height of your ascent.

4. Land on the balls of your feet, staying off heels.

5. Repeat for a set of eight, keeping ground contact short and your arms loose.

6. Rest for one minute.

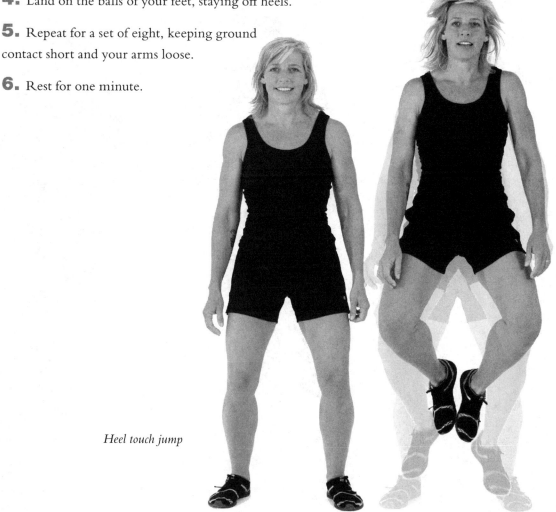

Heel touch jump

SIDE TO SIDE JUMPS

1. Start in your springiness position, again with your arms loose.

2. Shift your hips (your general center of mass) onto your right leg and drive off that leg, jumping to your left. This is a small jump, about six inches.

3. Land on the ball of your left foot, shifting your body weight to your left leg.

4. Repeat to the other side, driving off your left leg, for a set of eight. Keeping your upper body relaxed, try to center your hips over your support foot in each shuffle. Stay off your heels and keep ground contact short.

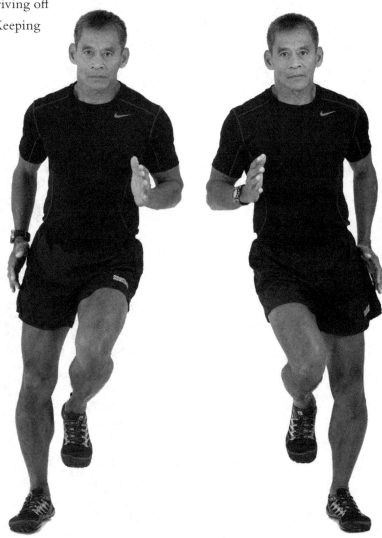

Side to side jumps

UPPING THE ANTE

As with all fitness activity, the more you do these exercises, the better you'll become. Your range of motion will improve week by week until your stretching poses look identical to the exemplary figures in the photographs. Each week, the number of jumping reps should increase from eight to ten to twelve to fifteen. What now seems unfamiliar and difficult will, a month from now, feel routine and accomplished. Most important, these improvements will mean you've built fitness foundation to make your transition to the right technique efficiently and without injury.

YOUR STRENGTH ROUTINE

Building Stability and Power

At the beginning of the running boom in the early 1970s, athletes and coaches dismissed strength training. The popular myth was it would make you muscle-bound. To get better at running, you simply ran. The focus was on the cardiovascular system—heart and lungs. They did not look at the body holistically. Basically they had one rule of thumb—high-volume training. Now leading scientists and coaches recognize the value of strength and conditioning as an essential component of a runner's repertoire.

The goal of this last preparatory chapter is to give you a running-specific strength routine to help you prevent injuries, run with proper technique, and achieve your running potential. You need to be strong enough to handle your body weight's interaction with gravity. In running, this load can increase from 1.5 times your body weight when jogging to 3 times your body weight when sprinting. If you weigh two hundred pounds, that means you need to make your body (muscles, tendons, ligaments, and bones) strong enough to handle loads from three hundred (jogging) to six hundred (sprinting) pounds. A body without a sufficient foundation of strength will not be able to perform and maintain proper technique.

Don't be daunted: This program will give you the strength you need to handle these demands. Just as you will complete the movement preparation sequence of the previous chapter before each and every workout, you will conclude each session with a strength routine. The exercises outlined below will tide you over for the next four weeks as you work your way through the ten lessons. Just like the jump routine in the previous chapter, the number of reps for each exercise will increase every week or so, as you'll see when you get to the lessons. Then, in about four weeks, when you reach the running circuit part of the Pose Method program, you'll encounter more challenging variations of these exercises.

Now it's time to become acquainted with the exercises you'll be doing every day. You'll want to keep these tips in mind:

- Initiate all of the movements from your hips.
- Keep your hips stable (glutes locked) and don't let them rotate or swivel to the left or right. For the plank moves, if being on your hands puts too much pressure on your wrists or is too difficult, you can support yourself on your forearms and elbows.
- Exhale when you're raising your hips and inhale when you're lowering your hips.
- Maintain good alignment, so that a straight line could be drawn from the ball of your foot through your hip and shoulder joint to your head—what I call Pose alignment, as you'll learn in the next chapter.
- Draw your belly button toward your spine to activate your core.

FACE-UP HIP DIPS

1. Sit on the floor with your hands behind you and directly under your shoulders (palms down, fingers pointing away from your feet) and with your legs extended in front of you.

2. Raise your hips up as high as you can, while supporting your body weight on your hands and heels.

3. Return to the starting position and repeat for a set of ten. The number of reps for all of these exercises will increase each week as dictated in the lessons to come.

Face-up hip dips

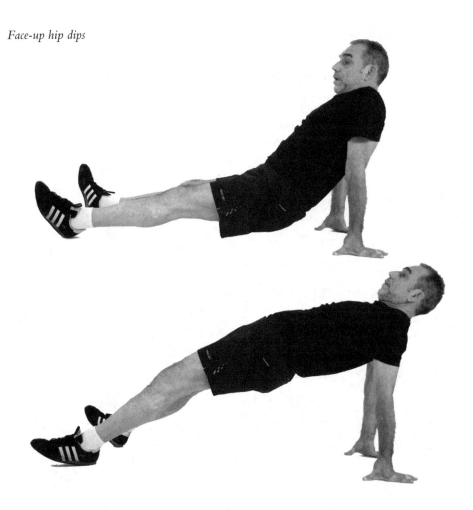

FACE-DOWN HIP DIPS

1. Assume a push–up position, with hands directly under your shoulders, arms extended, hips level with your body, and toes tucked.

2. Move the hips straight up in the air, making an upside–down V, similar to yoga's downward dog position.

3. Return to push-up position and repeat for a set of ten.

Face-down hip dips

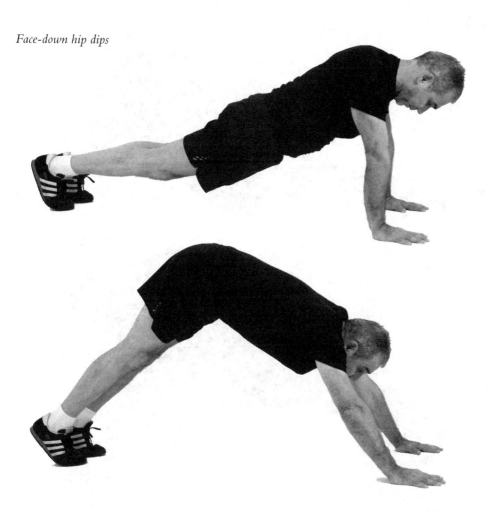

SIDE HIP DIPS

1. Get in a side plank position with your left arm extended and your left hand under your shoulder supporting your torso, hips resting on the ground.

2. Raise your hips straight up as high as you can.

3. Lower your hips back to the starting position and repeat for a set of ten.

4. Switch sides and complete ten more reps.

Side hip dips

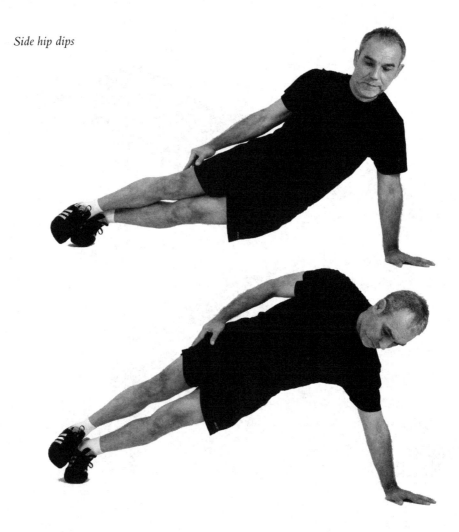

BODY WEIGHT SQUAT

1. Stand with your feet slightly wider than shoulder-width apart, hands extended straight ahead at shoulder level. Shift your body weight to the balls of your feet.

2. Lower your hips, sitting down and back as far as you can into a squatting position.

3. Return to the starting position and repeat for a set of ten.

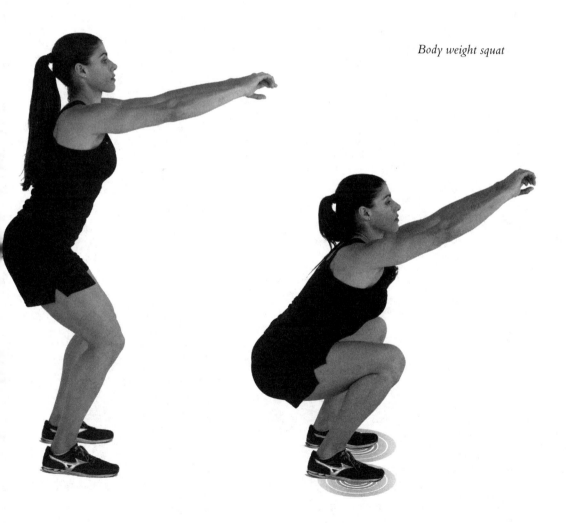

Body weight squat

PART TWO

TEN LESSONS

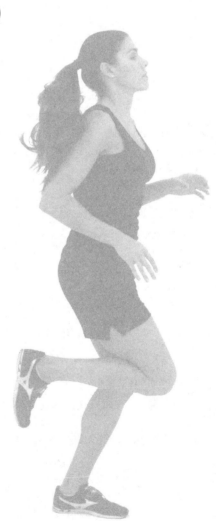

INTRODUCTION TO THE LESSONS

Mastering the Skill of Running

Forget any idyllic Garden of Eden of running when we ran barefoot and naked before Adam plucked a shoe with a built-up heel from the tree of running. In the early days, and still in some cultures, running happens uncorrupted by thick-heeled running shoes and a sedentary lifestyle. Now, in our modern world of bad habits, most of us have just as much to unlearn as we have to learn. So the idea of "just do it naturally" or "just do it" is not helpful advice. With running it's no longer natural to do it naturally. The following ten lessons ask you to let go of an ingrained movement pattern and replace it with a better one.

Like master classes, they are meant to be repeated again and again until perfection is attained. The movement preparation and strength training routines you learned in the previous chapters must accompany every session, even if you're already in great shape. Don't worry about forgetting to do them—you'll be reminded in each and every lesson. The goal is not to see how quickly you can breeze through the lessons. The goal of these master classes is to:

- Create new neurological patterns
- Build structural strength (muscles, tendons, and ligaments)
- Improve running biomechanics
- Create new perception of movement

This takes time, so be patient.

THE LESSON DESIGN

Each of the following ten lessons consists of a new key concept, an explanation of how this concept applies to proper running technique, a drill to inject this technique into your form, and a workout to help you practice and strengthen your improved form.

Each lesson begins with an introduction that provides both an overview and a look at the science and theory supporting the technique adjustments you'll be making. Here you'll learn which old rules about running no longer hold, and why.

The technique section will apply the lesson's key concept to a particular aspect of optimal running form. As I've said before, running naturally is a skill you must learn. In truth, it's an assembly of miniskills to be mastered one by one. In this section, the miniskill will be broken down and explained to you before you apply it to your form.

In the drill section you'll move from theory to practice, taking the concept and technique into the mechanics of your own running. This is the section that gets you off your butt and moving. You'll start with the movement preparation sequence outlined in part one, then embark on the drill set of the lesson. Once you've gotten the knack of each drill, you'll move on to the workout.

The workout combines drills and running with the goal of gradually shifting your form into Pose Method. Your practice sessions are progressive. In the beginning the workouts may seem ridiculously easy, but by lesson ten your workout is quite a bit longer. Enjoy the relative physical ease of the short early sessions, channeling your energy into the difficult mental task of rethinking your movement. You'll need to be tuned in as you constantly ask: Is my foot landing properly? Am I forcing it back down or just letting it fall? Am I relaxed, tensed, bouncing, or driving forward? This is a lot of information for the mind to process in a constructive way that avoids negative criticism and frustration at not achieving perfection right away.

Each workout will conclude with your strengthening routine—including information on the number of reps for that workout—and a running journal entry. You'll also be reminded when to break out the camera for an update on how your form looks on film.

SCHEDULING THE LESSONS

To follow a training program that matches your fitness level and fits your schedule, you need to make appointments with yourself. This requires:

- A running schedule for the week
- A specific workout time for each training day
- A multiweek calendar that can be adjusted as expectations develop and change

Now's the time to break out your calendar and running journal and lay out the first block of your Pose Method plan. You should devote at least two days to each new lesson, so if you're working out six days a week, you'll complete the ten lessons in no less than four weeks. Six days a week is a pretty intense schedule, but at this stage your workouts will be short in length and not intense, so you won't be breaking down your muscles. The frequency at this phase is to help you create a new movement pattern. If you've got the time, devotion, and strength to tackle the lessons at optimum pace, here's how you'll lay out your training plan in your journal:

- Week one: lessons 1–3
- Week two: lessons 4–6
- Week three: lessons 7–9
- Week four: lesson 10 and a review of the two lessons that were the most challenging

Each lesson session—including reading, movement preparation, drills, workout, and strength training—will average about thirty minutes, so in your calendar you'll want to book appointments with yourself accordingly. (The session time will increase after you finish the lessons and your running mileage increases.) If you can, you should let this month be about learning this new technique and not add running on top of it. If you're an avid runner, a break from your normal routine will be a positive. If you're just a beginner, you're not logging a lot of miles anyway.

Of course, not everyone will progress in a strict paint-by-the-numbers fashion. Some will progress at a steady pace while others will need to spend more time on certain lessons. This will mean setting aside a little extra time on a drill that is challenging, while still moving forward to the next lesson. If it takes you longer than one month to complete the lessons with a degree of mastery, then give yourself an extra week, adjusting your planner and noting any difficulties or hurdles in your journal.

In addition to your workout appointments, you should also schedule a reward system. If your training is a torture day after day without relief in sight, you'll quit. If you have a light at the end of the tunnel waiting for you after a particularly difficult lesson or workout sequence, you'll pull through. It can be as simple as a favorite treat at the end of your workout (a smoothie), your favorite meal on Friday (pizza), or buying yourself a new gadget at the three-month mark (an iPad).

Most important, don't be too gung-ho or greedy, wanting everything at once. Working out is for a lifetime. These lessons are just the beginning.

LESSON ONE

The Foot

Back in the day, hunters and gatherers didn't have Nike shoes. They developed moccasins, huaraches, and sandals with thin, flexible soles to protect the feet. It was minimal footwear, without big, built-up heels so they moved in harmony with the body's design.

A simple way to get a sense of how people ran before the running shoe explosion of the 1970s is to take off your shoes and run ten or twenty meters. It becomes clear that landing on your heel is painful and inefficient and landing on the ball of your foot feels good and makes sense. This doesn't mean you have to run barefoot all the time. It's to illustrate how optimal biomechanics (i.e., how your body moves) supports your body's structure and does not work against it. In this lesson we'll explore the foot's structure and function.

I don't want you to develop a foot fetish, but the structure of the foot is a miraculous and beautiful example of how form meets function. The human foot has 26 bones, 33 joints, 107 ligaments, 19 muscles, and 38 tendons. The 52 bones that make up your feet are about 25 percent of all the bones in your body. This complex matrix of muscles, tendons, ligaments, joints, and bones is your body's shock absorbing system. In this lesson we'll look at this elegant system as it relates to running.

As the triumphal arches of ancient Rome attest, there is no structure more resilient and supportive than the arch. The arch structure causes weight to move outward and downward, decreasing the load over space. This is the design nature gave to your foot. But your arches, unlike the Roman bridges, can do double duty; they support the load of your body weight and collapse to help reduce the impact of landing. They also have a built-in spring action that both decreases the impact of landing by compressing (coiling), and releases this potential energy into motion by expanding (springing). If you land on your heel, you deprive yourself of this spring system. In fact, you pervert the body's structure, using the old-fashioned definition of the word "pervert," which means to turn away from what is good or true. Instead of propelling you into your next stride with a *springlike* boost, the heel strike momentarily screeches on the brakes. Longtime USA Track & Field coach Rodney Wiltshire once explained why the heel strike is inefficient in very simple terms: "Biomechanically, when you heel strike you're literally putting on the brakes. Great runners don't put on the brakes with every stride."

How your body wants you to run is also revealed in the bones of your feet. The toe bones (phalanges) and larger bones that make up the bridge of the foot (the metatarsals) vary in thickness. The biggest and thickest of these bones by far is the big toe bone and the metatarsal bone that connects to the big toe. Big bones got big over time because they had to bear more weight. These big bones adapted and thickened to handle the stress and heavy load. Not following the wisdom of this design and the associated movement pattern will usually lead to injury (and inefficient movement). Your smaller toes function to increase your awareness (and perception) of your foot's position. They are not meant to take the impact of landing.

You do lead with your heel when you walk, because walking doesn't have the impact of running, the stride length of running, or anything resembling a flight phase.

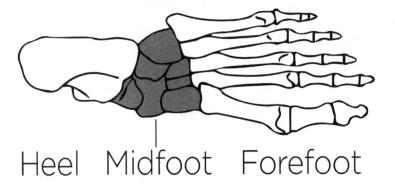

Heel Midfoot Forefoot

The human foot has twenty-six bones and can be broken down into three parts

TECHNIQUE: THE FOREFOOT LANDING DECONSTRUCTED

There's a lot of chatter in the running community not just about the best foot strike, but even about how to define these terms. Sometimes the forefoot landing and the midfoot landing are used interchangeably; sometimes they are given different definitions. Before we focus on the one and only landing endorsed in this book—the forefoot landing—let's define all three:

- Heel Strike: Landing on your heel first.
- Midfoot Strike: Landing simultaneously and with equal weight on

Heel strike

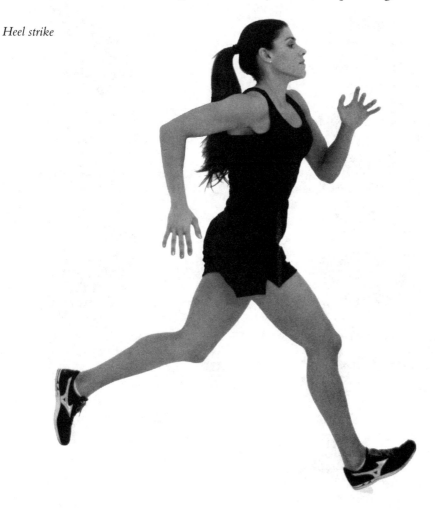

your heel and the ball of your foot. Sometimes this is called flat-foot landing. In Pose Method clinics we call this the unicorn landing because video analysis would say this rarely happens, even though runners claim this is the case. (Cue earlier discussion about perception.)

• Forefoot Landing: Landing on the balls of your feet.

Let me repeat: The forefoot landing is the only natural landing for a runner. No matter how you land, falling forward only happens after we shift onto our fore-

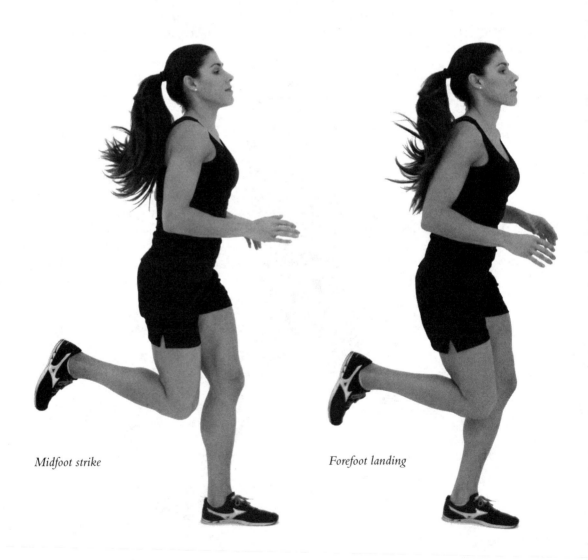

Midfoot strike   *Forefoot landing*

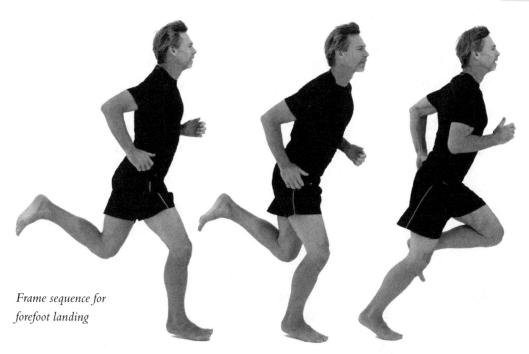

*Frame sequence for
forefoot landing*

*Natural angle of foot just
prior to ground contact*

foot. So the question is simple: Why postpone a necessary element of running with a deviation like heel striking when
we can land directly into our next point of action without
delay? Like most movements, we can break it down into a
sequence of frames, as in a filmstrip.

Beginning Frame: As the foot gets ready to make
contact with the ground it slightly supinates (the outside edge
of the foot angles toward the ground and the big toe elevates
slightly toward twelve o'clock).

Middle Frame: When contact with the ground is
made, the foot rolls inward, pronating toward the big toe as
the spring system coils. (Yes, a little bit of supination and pro-
nation is part of a natural foot landing. In the next illustration, you can see the ball of the foot is tilted at a sideways
angle.)

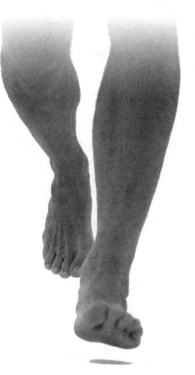

End Frame: The spring uncoils and body weight unloads over the ball of the foot and the big toe.

The Takeaway: Besides absorbing the shock of your body weight, landing on the ball of the foot unleashes the muscular-tendon elastic system, decreasing both impact and energy expenditure, while helping propel you into your next stride. The heel strike, by contrast, takes this beautifully evolved system out of the equation and the ankle, knee, and hip have to handle the impact of running. The result: an unacceptably high rate of injury.

DRILLS: BODY WEIGHT PERCEPTION

Body weight placement on the different parts of your feet reveals your mind-set—your attitude and desires toward the world. If you are on your heels, you are an old person because you don't want to move, and your physiology reflects this mind-set. If you are on the balls of your feet, you are a young person. You are ready and want to move, and your physiology will reflect these desires.

The goal of these drills is to help you develop perception of your body weight as it shifts to different parts of your feet. In the Focus Preparation segment of your journal entry, note that you will be exploring how to apply your body weight and how the feet help unload it. You generally don't have to think about all this—your foot does it for you—but a conscious exploration of the body weight mechanics at work will give you deep insight into your built-in spring system for support and returning kinetic energy to your moving body. Continue thinking about your body weight as you complete your movement preparation routine. Try to be mindful of how your muscles, bones, tendons, and ligaments are bearing and moving your weight.

Body Weight Perception Drill 1

The goal is to increase perception of where you feel body weight in your feet. Ultimately, you should be able to detect quick and subtle shifts.

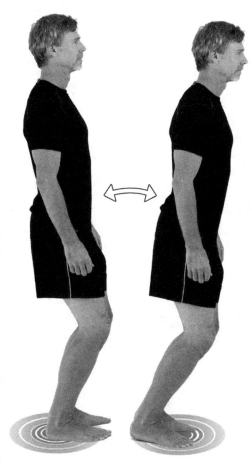

Body weight perception

1. With your shoes off, assume the springiness position, feeling a readiness in your body to move in any direction.

2. Slowly move your body weight around your feet, from front to back, from side to side, and in circular motion (like the hand around a clock).

3. Now narrow the placement of your body weight to specific spots of pressure in your feet:

  A. The balls of your feet

  B. Your heels

  C. Equal weight on heels and balls

  D. The outer edges of your feet

  E. The insides of your feet

4. Restore weight to the optimum position: the balls of your feet.

5. Repeat, gradually increasing the speed of these weight shift movements.

Body Weight Perception Drill 2

1. With your shoes off, assume springiness position: Your body is ready to move in any direction.

2. Begin running gently in place, feeling the spring action in your feet and registering each landing.

3. Note which part of your foot makes contact—heel, midfoot, forefoot? (Almost everyone lands on the balls of their feet when they run in place. If you're landing on your heels, call 911.)

4. Where in relation to the rest of your body does your foot make contact? Directly under your body? In front of it? Behind it?

5. Follow the sensation of each landing all the way up your body: ankles, knees, hips.

6. Perceive your whole body in space: your alignment, your running posture, and how it changes or stays the same in the different phases. Are your shoulders rounded? What's your head position?

7. Shift the position of your upper body: vertical, bending forward, bending backward. Register which position feels optimal for running.

WORKOUT

This workout is not physically challenging. It's all about getting in touch with your feet. You can repeat it any time you feel like you need to re-center and get back in touch with your body weight and readiness.

1. Complete the focus preparation segment in your journal.

2. Shift from your normal everyday standing posture to your springiness position. Check alignment. Continue to practice this shift until the springiness position is precise and intuitive. Repeat this shift a minimum of five times.

3. Complete both of the body weight perception drills at least three times every day you devote to Lesson One. You can do the first one when you are standing in line or just have a few spare moments.

4. Recruit a friend to capture you on film.

5. Go for a short run, one to two minutes, recording your form on video.

6. For your strength routine, do eight reps each for every exercise.

7. Complete a post-session review in your running journal. Don't stress out about being profound every time you sit down to write, but make sure you jot down a few thoughts about the session. This is also the best time to write down goals for your next workout. Review them as a way to prep for that session.

LESSON TWO

The Running Pose

In this lesson you'll be introduced to the running Pose. The other two frames are built out of this frame. As mentioned earlier, a frame is just like a film frame that captures a key moment in a dynamic sequence. It's an instant in time.

With the concept of the running Pose we depart from conventional thinking that says there is no universal pattern to optimum running, that sees running as an individual style, whereby everyone runs the way that feels best to him or her—heel strike or no. Conversely, I argue that there is a universal biomechanical structure to running. The running Pose is one of the three *invariable* elements of running—the foundational elements that every human body passes through when running. These elements are the running Pose, falling, and pulling. Great runners do it efficiently and average runners don't do it as well, but we all do it when we run. The three filmstrips on the following page show, frame by frame, how elite runners and recreational runners moving at three different speeds—fast, medium, slow—all pass through the running Pose. In each filmstrip the Pose frame is highlighted. You can see that no matter the speed or the expertise of the runner, they all move through the running Pose.

The running Pose is the moment when your full

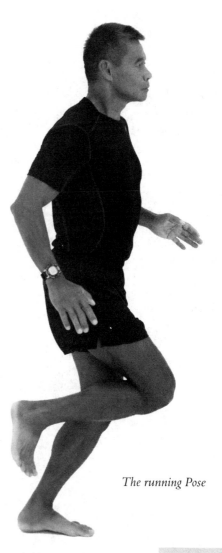

The running Pose

89

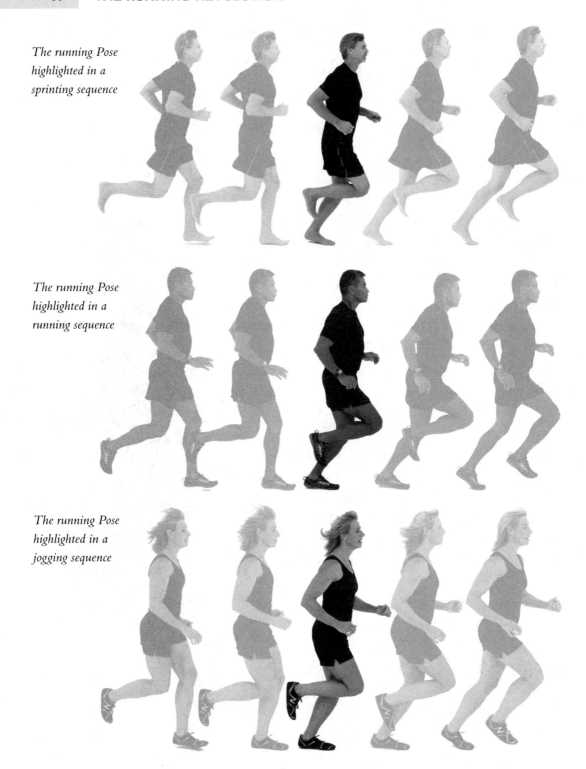

*The running Pose
highlighted in a
sprinting sequence*

*The running Pose
highlighted in a
running sequence*

*The running Pose
highlighted in a
jogging sequence*

body weight, combined with the increased load created by the speed of your running, meets the ground. This position is the same as your springiness position, except it is on one leg, and it represents your body's maximum energy potential for accelerating, like a ball on the edge of a table or at the top of a hill. Stability and alignment in this position are essential if you want to maximize that potential.

TECHNIQUE: GETTING INTO THE RUNNING POSE

1. Get in your springiness position.

2: Pull your right foot up under your hip, so your right ankle is level with your left knee, making the shape of the number four with your lower body.

3. Raise your left arm to counterbalance.

4. On your support leg, shift weight to the ball of your foot, with your heel still lightly touching the ground.

5. Bend the knee of your support leg so it is directly over your toes.

6. Flex your supporting hip slightly—it should be directly above the ball of your foot, while your shoulders are directly above your hips.

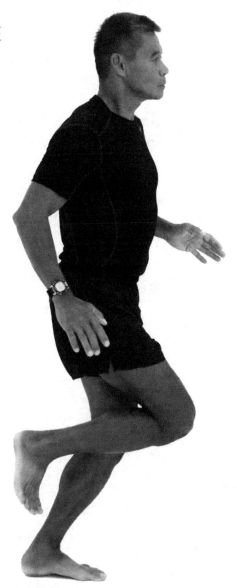

Getting into the running Pose

If you are in the proper running Pose, a straight line could be drawn from the ball of your supporting foot through the hip and shoulder joint to the head. You should feel poised to fall, even desiring to fall—the reasons for this are set forth in the next lesson. For now, you'll simply have to trust me.

DRILLS: THE RUNNING POSE

The goal of these drills is to ingrain the Pose position into your mind and body by increasing the perception of where you feel the body weight in your feet, and by cultivating balance. Ultimately, you should be able to detect quick and subtle shifts without varying your position much at all.

Body Weight Perception in the Running Pose Drill

1. Get into the running Pose.

2. Feel the pressure on the ball of your foot, noting how the running Pose feels different from standing on two legs. Do you feel any weak links in your alignment chain?

3. Shift pressure around your support foot: your toes, your heel, with equal weight on the heel and ball, with weight on the outside of your foot, with weight on the inside of your foot. Which muscles do you feel being activated with each shift?

4. Now place your body weight back in the optimum position on the ball of your foot.

5. Switch the support foot and repeat, noting whether one leg feels different from the other.

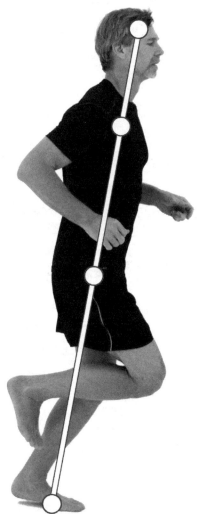

In the running Pose, a straight line can be drawn from the ball of the support foot through the hip and shoulder joint to the head.

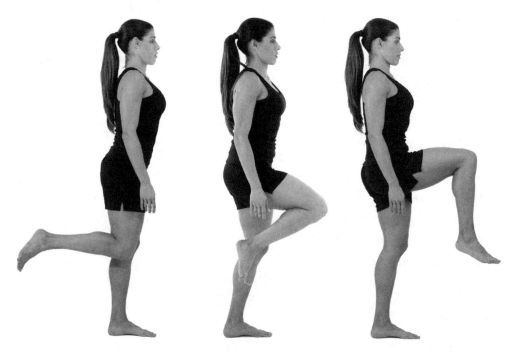

Pose Hold Drill

The middle photo illustrates the proper position of the leg for the running Pose.

1. Get in the running Pose.

2. Check to make sure you're not pulling behind you, or raising your knee out in front. The correct running Pose (middle illustration) is with the foot underneath the hip.

3. Feel the pressure on the ball of your foot.

4. Hold the running Pose for ten to twenty seconds, using balance rather than muscular effort to keep pressure on the ball of your foot. If you lose balance, gently bring pressure back to the ball of your foot.

5. Repeat with the other leg.

WORKOUT

The goal of this lesson's workout is to develop the strength and coordination to maintain proper running Pose. Don't move on to Lesson Three before you've mastered the position and can complete all three sets with ease.

1. Complete the focus preparation segment of your running journal.

2. Work up to three sets of Pose holds, focusing your perception on key points of your power position: the ball of your foot, the slight bend in your joints. Check alignment from foot to head to develop an intuitive feel for the running Pose. Maintain the intention of movement, of falling forward, even though you are working on a static hold.

3. Go for a short run, one to two minutes, and try to replicate the running Pose each time you land.

4. For your strength routine, do eight reps each for every exercise.

5. Complete the post-session review in your running journal, recording your observations about your experience with the running Pose. How did it feel different from simply standing on two legs? Did you struggle to maintain balance and alignment? Which muscles felt strongest, and which the weakest, when you shifted pressure around your foot and when you held the Pose position? What are your goals for your next training session?

LESSON THREE

Falling

No matter how wild this may sound, natural running is just free falling. You fall and catch yourself over and over. The key to falling—without collapsing—is to utilize the power of gravity to drive your movement forward.

Gravity affects every move you make. Without gravity, you'd float off into the atmosphere. Every time you jump, you experience gravity. It pulls you back down to the ground in a vertical line, just like when you drop a ball. When you fall forward, gravity is the downward force vector acting on your body's torque—arguably the most crucial physics concept at the heart of the Pose Method.

Gravitational torque happens when your hips (your general center of mass) move past your support foot (your axis of rotation, in physics speak). Imagine a bowling pin balanced on the ground. If you slowly push it forward, there will be a moment when its general center of mass will travel beyond its base of support and it will fall forward—not because of your lateral push, but because of the downward force of gravity now acting upon the bowling pin's center of mass. Your ability to utilize gravitational torque—to fall forward—is the key to fast, efficient running.

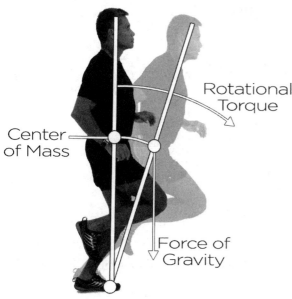

A runner's gravitational torque

This assertion runs against the conventional thinking that a runner's speed and forward locomotion are the products of active leg extension and knee drive—muscular activity long considered to trigger the propulsive drive phase of running.

Enter a team of researchers at Penn State University (McClay, Lake, and Cavanagh), who in 1990 confronted this assumption head-on. They used electromyography sensors to test muscle activation during running. The definitive results of their study revealed that the extensor muscles (major quad muscles in the thigh) were *not* active during the drive phase of running. These were muscles the researchers had assumed would be the *most* active during ground push off, and instead they were actually shutting off. Many a head was scratched in confusion: The study's indisputable results didn't fit into the accepted paradigm of driving with the legs in running, so the result of the study was labeled the extensor paradox. The very name illustrates how it has left sports scientists and coaches perplexed for over twenty years.

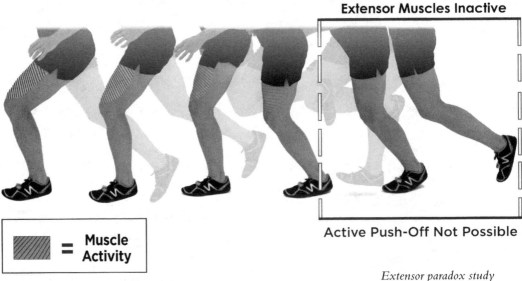

Extensor paradox study

But for me and other students of the Pose Method, this research did not cause any confusion. It did just the opposite. The Penn State study confirmed my theory that gravity is the most efficient and powerful force for forward movement. So when you start to fall out of the running Pose, the body automatically turns off the quadriceps. Your own body weight and the angle of your falling—your torque— provide forward propulsion, cueing your quad muscles to shut down, as electromyography data show.

TECHNIQUE: HOW TO FALL

Falling is not easy. You have to overcome a movement pattern and a notion that is deeply ingrained in your body: that you push off the ground to move forward when you run. As you complete your movement preparation sequence, think about all the patterns embedded in the muscles that propel you forward when you run. As you move your joints through a full range of motion and relax

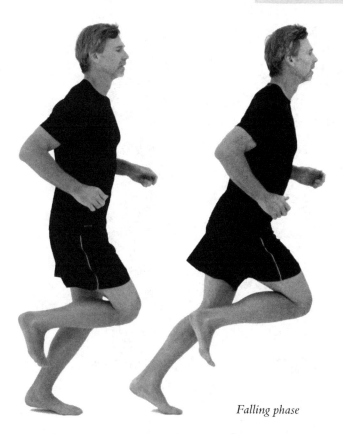

Falling phase

your muscles during the flexibility routine, try to imagine how these muscles are engaged when you run. You are about to revolutionize those patterns with a new way of running.

Here's the new way:

1. Get in your springiness position.

2. Maintaining alignment, begin to move your hips (your general center of mass) forward over the balls of your feet (your point of support). There will be a tipping point when your hips pass the balls of your feet, your heels will come off the ground, and you will begin falling. Focus on letting go of stabilization muscles that are helping you maintain balance and fall forward in a free fall. Let your entire body fall as one unit.

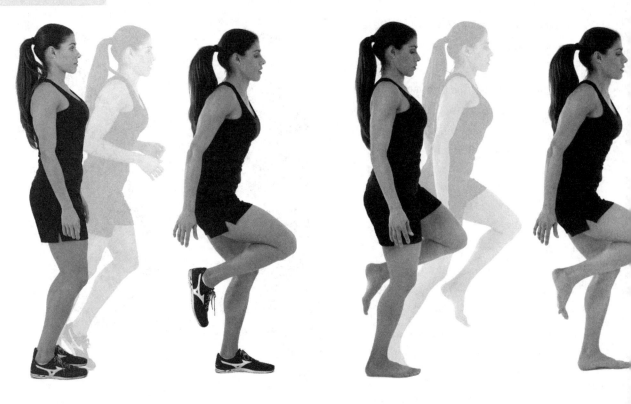

Free fall into the running Pose   *Free fall in the running Pose and change of support*

3. Now you have two choices as gravity takes over: Fall on your face or bring one of your legs forward to catch yourself. I recommend bringing a leg forward. It's like the trust game when you fall backward and your partner catches you, not letting you crash to the ground, but in this case you catch yourself.

4. Follow the same procedure, but from the running Pose. Have your body fall as one single unit in the running Pose over your point of support (the ball of your foot), so you maintain your postural line as you fall. Try to increase your perception of falling and letting go.

DRILLS: FALLING

These falling drills are about perception. You have to let go of the idea of using muscles to drive yourself forward and give in to the idea of the free fall.

Springiness Position Wall-Fall Drill

1. Get in your springiness position. Stand about three feet from a wall, facing the wall.

2. Prepare to fall.

3. Fall, by moving your hips forward over your point of support, the balls of your feet. Maintain your springiness position as you fall forward and keep your ankles loose.

4. Catch yourself with your hands. When you land, your hips should remain stable and should not continue moving forward. When the upper body stops falling forward, your hips must stop, too.

5. Repeat until you are comfortable letting go and falling.

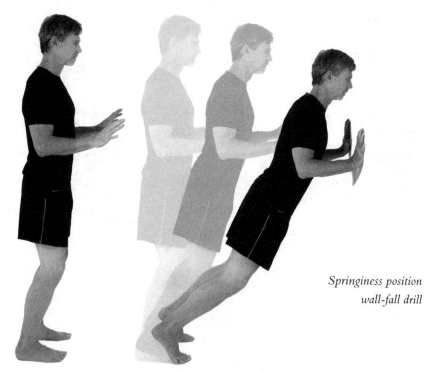

*Springiness position
wall-fall drill*

The Running Pose Wall-Fall Drill

1. Assume the running Pose. Stand about three feet from a wall, facing the wall.

2. Prepare to fall. Extend your arms at shoulder level to stop your fall.

3. Fall by moving your hips forward over your point of support, the balls of your feet. Maintain your running Pose as you fall forward and keep your support ankle loose.

4. Catch yourself with your hands. Remember that when the upper body stops falling forward, the hips must stop, too.

5. Repeat with the other leg as your support leg.

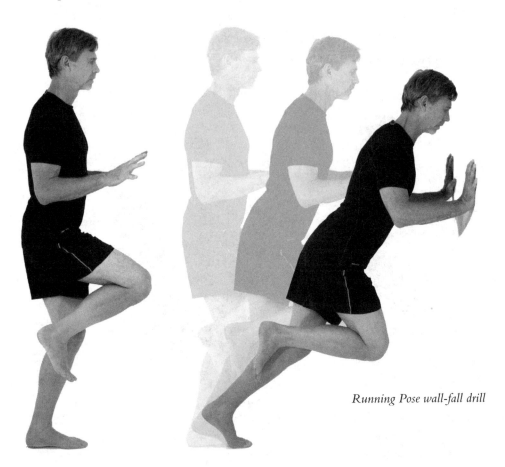

Running Pose wall-fall drill

Timber Drill

1. Get into the running Pose.

2. Let your body fall forward like a tree—timber! As always, maintain the running Pose as you fall forward, keeping your support ankle loose.

3. Catch yourself with your nonsupport foot, landing on the ball of your foot with your hips stable. They should not continue moving forward.

4. Pull the other foot into the running Pose.

5. Repeat with the other leg.

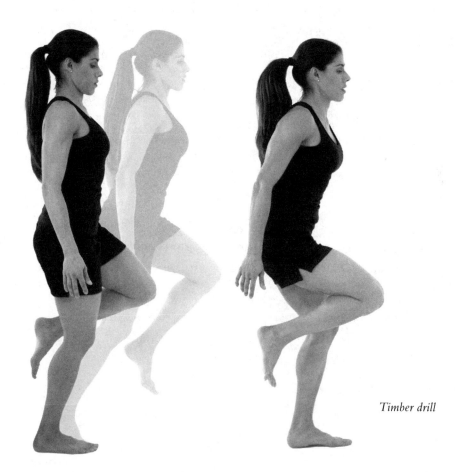

Timber drill

WORKOUT

The Lesson Three workout is all about getting the feeling of falling ingrained in your body. Consistency is the key, and to accomplish this you will be reviewing all the drills you've mastered in the previous lessons as well as Lesson Three. From now on, each lesson's workouts will include a cumulative set of drills.

1. Complete the Focus Preparation segment of your running journal.

2. Complete all three body weight perception drills—springiness position, running in place, and Pose position.

3. Do the Pose hold drill for twenty seconds on each leg, for a set of three.

4. Complete three reps of the wall-fall drill from the springiness position, and three reps on each leg from the running Pose. As you become more comfortable falling, move farther away from the wall to make the drill more challenging.

5. Complete three timber drill reps on each support leg from the running Pose.

6. Go for a short run, one to two minutes, and try to land in the Pose with each step. You'll need to consciously work on your desire to fall every time you run.

7. For your strength routine, do eight reps for every exercise.

8. Complete the post-session review in your running journal, recording your observations about the art of falling forward. Did you maintain the integrity of the running Pose as you fell forward and made ground contact? Did you land on the ball of your foot? Did you allow falling to truly be the cause of landing on the ball of your foot? What are your goals for your next training session?

LESSON FOUR

The Pull

In this lesson you'll enter the phase that sets running apart from walking: the flight phase, when both feet are off the ground. While conventional thinking has dictated that the force that drives a runner forward into the flight phase requires *pushing* off the ground, I maintain that the natural way to run requires just the opposite. You accomplish flight by *pulling* your support foot off the ground at the end of the falling phase, before your lead foot lands again in the running Pose. You pull into Pose to fall, to pull again. Pose is pull's target.

There are several mechanisms at work to break contact with the ground and get us into the flight phase. The first one is the elasticity or recoiling effect, which is produced by an unweighing action (swinging action) of the shoulders, arms, and swing leg. The second happens during falling forward, when the pressure on the ground dissipates as the body weight shifts off support.

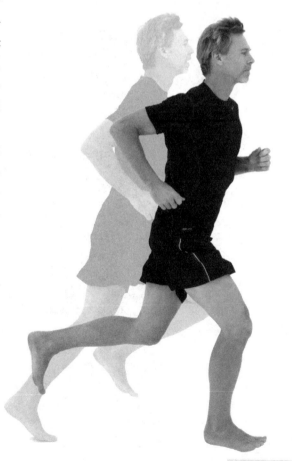

The pull phase

TECHNIQUE

Pulling is simply the action of raising your support foot off the ground directly under your hip, ideally when your nonsupport leg swings past your support leg and begins its descent toward the ground to catch your fall. This action launches you into the flight phase, when both legs are off the ground.

Here's the basic sequence for the pulling leg:

1. Keeping it in a neutral position (not pointed up or down), bring your foot up directly under your hip, not in front or behind it.

2. As you continue falling forward, maintaining Pose alignment, this foot naturally swings through to catch you.

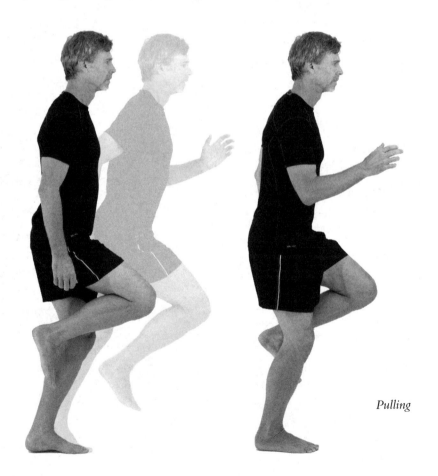

Pulling

CHANGE OF SUPPORT DRILL

This is a challenging drill because you're being asked to change support from one leg to another from a stationary position. When you're running you have the help of gravity (falling) and momentum to help you change support into your next stride. The goal of all the drills is to present challenges that build your perception and your muscles to improve your running. So the drills are not exactly the same as running, just like practicing scales on the piano is not the same as playing a Bach composition, but practicing the scales helps. In the beginning, if you struggle with this drill, you can slightly bend the knee in your support leg to load the joint and muscles to help you initiate the pulling movement. Do this one foot at a time, concentrating on centering your body weight on the ball of the foot when you land. (Don't simply run in place!)

Change of support drill

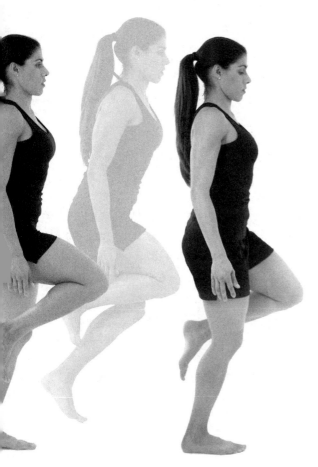

1. Start in the running Pose on your left leg, focusing on how you will be lifting your left foot off the ground and under the hip before the other foot drops.

2. Swing your right leg forward as you fall.

3. When your right foot passes your left leg, lift your left foot up under your hip while the right foot is still in the air, shifting your weight toward your right leg to catch yourself. As you change support, lift your shoulders to help unload body weight.

4. Letting your right leg naturally drop to the ground with no muscular effort, land on the ball of your foot in perfect Pose position.

5. Repeat with your other leg, pulling the right foot up under your hip, shifting your weight, and landing on your left foot in perfect Pose position.

WORKOUT

1. Complete the focus preparation segment of your running journal.

2. Complete all three body weight perception drills—springiness position, running in place, and the running Pose.

3. Do the Pose hold drill for twenty seconds on each leg, for a set of three.

4. Complete three reps of the wall-fall drill from the springiness position, and three reps on each leg from the running Pose, moving farther away from the wall to challenge yourself.

5. Complete three timber drill reps on each support leg from the Pose position. For variety, raise your nonsupport foot to different levels in relation to your support foot: ankle, midcalf, knee.

6. Complete ten change of support drill reps, resting thirty seconds between each.

7. Go for a short run (one to two minutes), focusing on the pull and feeling the new movement pattern in your body.

8. For your strength routine, increase your volume to ten reps of each exercise.

9. Complete the post-session review in your running journal, recording your observations about your success with the pull phase of running. Did your support leg leave the ground, pulling upward, before your other foot dropped toward the ground? Did you let your airborne leg drop to the ground with no muscular effort (letting gravity do all the work)? How did you overcome inertia (with no help from gravity or momentum) to change support? What are your goals for your next training session?

LESSON FIVE

Integrating the Frames

In the past, when you thought about a run, you probably thought about your route, how far and how fast. Then, during the run, you let the noise in your head take over—work, dinner, relationship issues, et cetera. Or you plugged in your iPod. But as I mentioned much earlier in this book, in order to master a new method, you need to tune in to your running process. In this lesson you'll get specific things to focus your mind on continuously as you run.

ANATOMY OF A STRIDE

Traditionally, running has been defined by the work of Geoffrey Dyson as support, drive, and recovery. Conversely, the Pose paradigm for running is: Pose, fall, pull. For the past several lessons, you've been learning this technique one element at a time. Now it's time to put it all together.

The illustration below covers various running elements frame by frame, both the invariable elements that all runners move through and the variable inefficiencies that many runners add as they stride along.

Anatomy of a stride

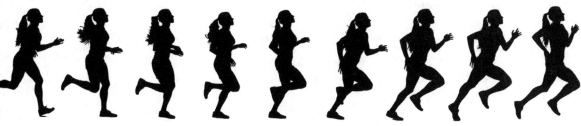

| Heel Strike | Midfoot Strike | Forefoot Strike | Paw Back | Running Pose | Falling Forward | Knee Drive | Push Off | Pulling |

1. **Heel Strike:** You can heel strike, but it's not your optimal position for landing and it's the major cause of injury for various reasons: higher incidence of oversupination and overpronation; locked joints in the ankle, knee, and hip; longer support time on the ground.

2. **Midfoot Strike:** Better than a heel strike—if you are indeed achieving the elusive midfoot landing—but it still results in your foot landing ahead of your body, which produces excess knee strain and has a braking effect on your momentum.

3. **Forefoot Strike:** The preferred landing of the Pose Method, which distributes the force of impact into your muscles and tendons instead of locked joints, resulting in minimal support time on the ground and maximum elasticity in your legs.

4. **Paw Back:** This concept comes from the field of sprinting; it's mechanically impossible to achieve and results in hitting the ground harder than necessary, potentially leading to injury.

5. **Running Pose:** You will at some point in your stride be in the running Pose—ideally on your forefoot—no matter how poor or masterful your technique is.

6. **Falling:** Whether you waste energy by pushing yourself off the ground or conserve energy by letting gravity do its work on your body, this is another invariable aspect of every runner's form. Ideally, you will fall forward to move forward.

7. **Knee Drive:** While many coaches have advised runners to drive the knee forward to maximize momentum, this actually slows down the general center of mass to compensate for the forward drive, straining the hip flexors and wasting muscle energy.

8. **Push Off:** Like the knee drive, pushing off wastes energy, increasing the runner's vertical movement but providing little forward momentum. Moreover, the muscles around the ankle that provide extension for push off are among the slowest in the body.

9. **Pulling:** Another phase that is invariably part of every runner's form, a well-timed pull at the correct position is your secret to running longer and faster.

TECHNIQUE

In order to put all the phases together—Pose, fall, and pull—into a smooth, efficient stride, you will need to hone your perception skills to perfection. But don't expect perfection at this stage. It's common to feel a little confused or even doubtful about the new techniques you're applying to your form. Old habits die hard. Let's return to the three running phases we first encountered at the beginning of this book. Below are the easy to identify visual markers of a stride. Study this graphic until these images form in your mind.

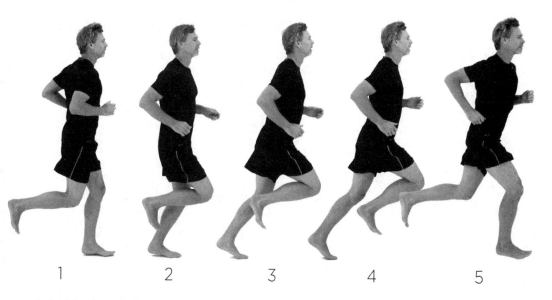

1   2   3   4   5

1. Initial contact. 2. Running Pose. 3. Heel lifts as the body begins falling. 4. Falling ends when the swing foot passes support leg and trail leg pulls up. 5. Flight phase.

MIND-BODY STRIDE DRILL

1. Run for thirty to sixty seconds, depending on your fitness level.

2. Walk for sixty seconds, asking yourself the following questions.

   • **How does my Pose frame feel?** Do I sense pressure on the ball of my support foot? Do I have my swing foot under my hip?

- **How does my falling frame feel?** Do I feel tension in my ankle? Do I feel an effortless movement forward through the sensation of falling? Do I feel this falling action leading to natural momentum like that of a ball rolling?

- **How does my pull frame feel?** Do I feel my swing foot being pulled directly up under my hip before my other foot lands?

3. If you are struggling with any of these three key elements, do a drill for that frame.

4. Move right into a thirty-second run.

5. Under a reframe headline in your journal, take specific notes on how you felt, focusing on positive critique:

- Did you have moments when the running felt light and effortless?

- Did you have a series of strides when you felt like you were doing everything technically right?

- What do you feel when you're doing well?

- What do you feel when you are struggling with form?

WORKOUT

Starting with this lesson, you'll be kicking it up a notch in the intensity and duration of your workout. In order to avoid injury and burnout, you need to keep a few points in mind.

First, this program is all about process, not performance. Everyone starts at a different level of fitness, so do what you can. Second, remember that it takes time to build up your mental habits. If your mind wanders, bring it back to your task. If your technique gets sloppy, walk for a longer period to get focused before you start running again. Third, and most important: If you get too tired, rest until you're recovered. If you feel like what you are doing is hurting you, then stop.

1. Complete the focus preparation segment of your running journal. Call up the three poses illustrated above, and write a few notes about how you will take them out with you for a run.

2. Complete all three body weight perception drills—springiness position, running in place, and the running Pose.

3. Do the Pose hold drill for twenty seconds on each leg, for a set of three.

4. Complete three reps of the wall-fall drill from the springiness position, and three reps on each leg from the running Pose, moving farther away from the wall to challenge yourself.

5. Complete three timber drill reps on each support leg from the running Pose, raising your nonsupport foot to different levels in relation to your support foot: ankle, midcalf, knee.

6. Complete ten change of support drill reps, resting thirty seconds between each.

7. Complete the mind-body stride drill, alternating thirty to sixty seconds of running with sixty seconds of walking for a total of ten minutes.

8. For your strength routine, do ten reps of each exercise.

9. Complete the post-session review in your running journal, recording your observations and feelings about the integration of the running Pose, falling, and pulling into your stride. Did you get tired or experience any pain? Did your mind wander or did you stay mentally focused? Reframe any frustrations you contended with. What are your positive takeaways? What are your goals for your next training session?

LESSON SIX

The Achilles Tendon

"Achilles" should be a happy word, not something we utter in fear. Forget the vulnerable mythological connotation. Your Achilles is *not* a fragile tendon, and its main function is *not* to help the foot push off in the drive phase—that is, unless you want to go down the road of Achilles tendonitis.

In truth, the main function of the Achilles, your body's biggest and most robust tendon, is to absorb the impact of landing and release energy back into your forward movement. Its long, elastic tissue connects the calf muscles to the heel bone, storing and releasing energy into each stride. It can easily support a lifetime of running if not misused.

In this lesson you'll learn how this relates to the forefoot landing, as well as about your Achilles' key role in helping you take advantage of a biomechanics phenomenon called ground reaction force.

Ground reaction force (GRF) happens when your foot makes contact with the ground and the ground pushes back with equal force. Think of it as the runner's version of Newton's Third Law: For every action there is an equal and opposite reaction. The greater your angle of falling, the greater your GRF. When your foot makes contact with the ground, your muscles and tendons lengthen like a bowstring, absorbing the GRF of impact. The muscles and tendons then shorten, releasing the absorbed energy back into your stride like an arrow released by a bow. Your Achilles tendon is at the root of this muscle-tendon elasticity system, which includes other tendons and ligaments, like a shock absorber spring and its attachments.

This only happens if you land on your forefoot. If you heel strike, not only do you lose the brilliant design of your body that helps you run, you also damage your body with a double impact on both your heel and forefoot. The heel impact is the most damaging because it uses your body like a hammer, coming down with full

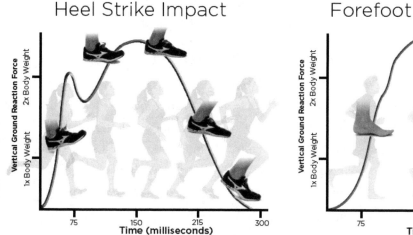

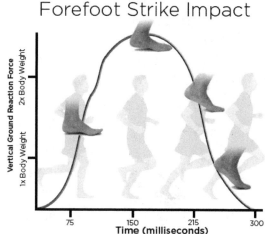

Ground reaction force: heel strike versus forefoot landing

impact all at once. The forefoot landing, on the other hand, is a slower absorption of the impact, then a *springlike* release into the next stride. This is represented by the graphic on the left, which illustrates the effects of a heel strike landing. The sharp spike represents the heel strike and the softer, rounded curve shows the forefoot strike.

In the world of exercise science, muscle-tendon elasticity is also called the stretch-shortening cycle. When the muscle-tendon elasticity system is effectively used to harness GRF, the energy cost of running can be reduced by 50 percent. In short, you will use less energy and perform better when you don't over-muscle your stride or heel strike.

TECHNIQUE: FOREFOOT LANDING REVISITED

In Lesson One you learned that to land in the proper running Pose, you must land on the ball of your foot with your ankle under your hip, rather than on your heel first with your foot well ahead of your hip. But in order to take full advantage of the GRF and the muscle-tendon elasticity system around your Achilles tendon, there are nuances to the forefoot landing that need to be worked into your technique.

Most important, you must remember that the forefoot landing is a consequence of falling, not an active strike of your foot against the ground. If you simply replace an active heel strike with an active forefoot strike, you will not decrease your chances of injury and you will not be running optimally. This is a common mistake among barefoot and minimalist shoe runners, who fall prey to the misconception that all will be corrected by simply landing on your forefoot.

One trick to making sure you are *landing* rather than *striking* is to avoid full extension of your joints. If you are landing in the proper running Pose, your support leg will form an S-shaped curve with your torso and head, and you will be less likely to strike the ground with your foot well in front of your body.

When you do land, the contact should be quick and quiet. As the Achilles stretches to absorb GRF, your heel should drop to touch the ground with a little kiss, while most of your body weight remains on the ball of your foot as the muscles and tendons shorten again and release your support foot for takeoff.

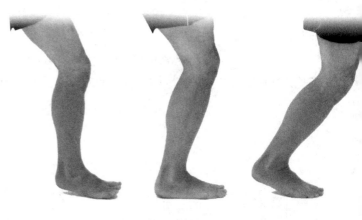

A runner's support foot at landing, midstance, and takeoff.

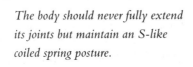

The body should never fully extend its joints but maintain an S-like coiled spring posture.

FOCUS PREPARATION:
IN SEARCH OF MY SWEET SPOT

The thing I've been trying to discover over the course of these lessons is what I think of as my sweet spot, the perfect landing and the perfect body position. The landing that feels like my foot and body are springs, so that when I land the impact is absorbing energy and releasing energy back into my movement.

When I hit my sweet spot I also utilize Newton's Third Law in the most efficient way—for every action there is an equal and opposite reaction. This is, for me, the running zone. It is all about technique, making running feel effortless with no wear and tear on my body.

BASE JUMP WITH FORWARD MOVEMENT DRILL

The goal is to increase your perception of falling forward and catching yourself as a way of harnessing ground reaction force.

1. Start in your springiness position.

2. Shift your hips (your center of gravity) over your base of support (your feet) and fall forward.

3. Jump to catch yourself, taking care not to push off from your toes or to use your calf muscles. This is different from doing a broad jump to see how far you can leap. The movement forward should come from falling forward, aided by a slight raising of your shoulders as you jump. The more severe your angle of

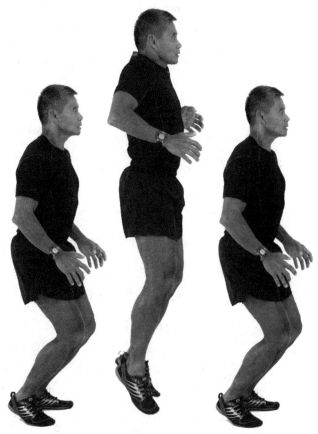

Base jump with forward movement drill

falling before you jump to catch yourself, the greater the forward distance you will cover.

4. Land on the balls of your feet, letting your heels kiss the floor.

5. Repeat for a series of jumps forward, making sure you can feel your body weight on the balls of your feet before you do your next forward jump.

WORKOUT

1. Complete the focus preparation segment of your running journal.

2. Complete all three body weight perception drills—springiness position, running in place, and the running Pose.

3. Do the Pose hold drill for twenty seconds on each leg, for a set of three.

4. Complete three reps of the wall-fall drill from the springiness position, and three reps on each leg from the running Pose, moving farther away from the wall to challenge yourself.

5. Complete three timber drill reps on each support leg from the Pose position, raising your nonsupport foot to different levels in relation to your support foot: ankle, midcalf, knee.

6. Complete ten change of support drill reps, resting thirty seconds between each.

7. Complete ten to twenty reps of the base jump with forward motion drill.

8. Alternate thirty to sixty seconds of running with sixty seconds of walking for a total of ten minutes, running through the frame questions of the mind-body stride drill. As you consider your Pose frame, can you feel your Achilles absorbing GRF and releasing energy back into your stride?

9. For your strength routine, complete ten reps of each exercise.

10. Complete the post-session review in your running journal, recording your observations and feelings of GRF in your forefoot, Achilles, and elsewhere throughout your body. Reframe any frustrations you contended with. Did you shift your hips (your center of gravity) over your base of support as you jumped? Did your movement come from falling forward? How did it feel to increase your angle of falling before jumping forward? Did you stick your landing, making contact with the balls of your feet, letting your heels kiss the floor? What are your goals for your next training session?

LESSON SEVEN

Pose Frame Revisited

In this lesson you'll take the entire Pose frame into motion, integrate shoulder and arm movements, and play with different speeds of running so that no matter how fast or far you're going, you'll learn to hit the running Pose with every step.

But first let's take down another long-held idea about running form: the role of the arms for acceleration. While conventional coaching dictates that the runner's shoulders should be kept down and back, and that the function of arm pumping is to increase speed, the Pose Method dictates that shoulders should be loose, rising and falling slightly, helping you unload body weight with each step. The function of the arms is to a create counterbalance to your legs.

Let's look at the runner as a mechanical system. In this system, there is a consistent flow of energy from the legs, through the trunk, and out into the arms. This flow, or transformation, of energy is significant for the physical balance of the body, and the arms play a vital role in maintaining this balance. This week you'll be increasing the number of jumps in your movement preparation routine from ten to fifteen. As you do this, pay close attention to the way your arms, trunk, and legs are interacting.

In the mechanical progression of running, the action starts with the act of falling forward, followed immediately by the rapid change of support from one leg to the next. As an automatic reaction to maintain balance, the body adds a slight rotation of the shoulder, opposite the leg giving up support, thus helping maintain balance. As the shoulders rotate, there is a corresponding movement of the arms.

In this sequence of movements, the arms are basically at the end of the line. In the hierarchy of this system, this means they do less work. It doesn't mean they are not important, but their actions must work in harmony with the system. If they try to do more work than the system needs, they destroy the efficiency and effectiveness of the movement.

The role of the arms, then, is to listen to the legs and body and be ready to react to any changes in their activity, by making the necessary adjustments to maintain balance. For example, if you stumble on a rough trail, the arms instantly and automatically make the adjustments to correct balance and assist you as you return to optimal form. Unless called upon in such a situation, the arms are always at the ready, doing as little as possible to maintain perfect form and balance.

This means specifically that you don't put them to work by exaggerated pumping, trying to speed them up to move faster than your legs, swinging them in front of your body or up to your shoulders. This will have a negative reciprocal effect on your trunk, causing it to move unnecessarily. At the same time you don't want to just let your arms dangle at your sides. You want them to move in opposition to your legs for counterbalance. The movement should be a natural rhythmic consequence of your speed and leg movements, not something you muscle or pump.

Now, about those legs . . .

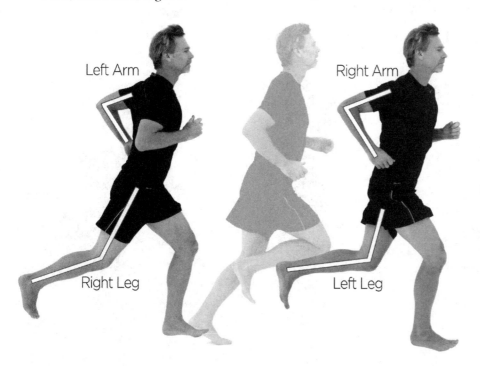

Natural rhythmic arm movement

TECHNIQUE: HITTING THE RUNNING POSE PERFECTLY EVERY TIME

To hit the running Pose precisely with each step, you need to be perceptive of counterbalancing with your arms and keeping your trunk upright, maintaining the S shape of your support leg and body. You maintain this S shape while you focus on shifting your body weight forward to your swing leg and landing on the ball of your foot under your hips every single step—all while cultivating the mental desire and readiness to fall.

CHANGE OF SUPPORT FORWARD MOTION DRILL

In lesson four you worked on change of support. Now it's time to take it into motion.

1. Start in the running Pose on your right leg.

2. Focus on changing support as you move your hips forward.

3. Fall forward, moving your hip over your point of support (the ball of your right foot).

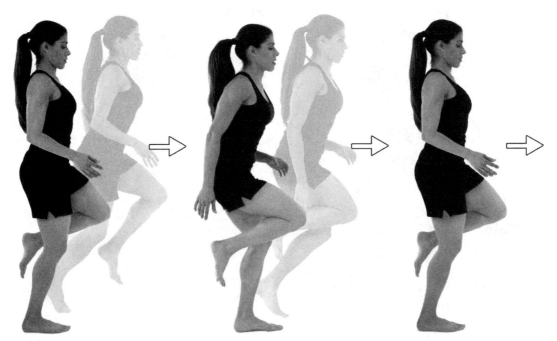

Change of support forward motion drill

4. Lift your shoulders to help unload body weight as you pull your right leg up under your hip, making sure your legs resemble the number 4 in profile.

5. Land on your left forefoot, letting your heel kiss the floor and then rise again as your muscle-tendon elasticity system stretches and recoils for release. Your hip should be directly above your support foot and your left leg should be bent slightly to form an S shape with your body.

6. As soon as you register your full body weight on the ball of your left foot, fall forward, shifting your body weight past the ball of your foot.

7. Pull your left foot up under your hip, using your right arm as a counterbalance as your support shifts toward your right foot.

8. Land on your right forefoot, with your hip directly above it and your right leg bent in the bottom half of an S shape.

9. Repeat the change of support, falling to move forward.

WORKOUT

1. Complete the focus preparation segment of your running journal.

2. Complete all three body weight perception drills—springiness position, running in place, and the running Pose.

3. Do the Pose hold drill for twenty seconds on each leg, for a set of three.

4. Complete three reps of the wall-fall drill from the springiness position, and three reps on each leg from the running Pose, moving farther away from the wall to challenge yourself.

5. Complete three timber drill reps on each support leg from the Pose position, raising your nonsupport foot to different levels in relation to your support foot: ankle, midcalf, knee.

6. Complete ten change of support drill reps, resting thirty seconds between each.

7. Complete ten to twenty reps of the base jump forward motion drill, rest for thirty to sixty seconds, and repeat for a total of two sets.

8. Engage in the change of support forward motion drill, stringing together as many strides as you can, until you experience a breakdown in technique or you run out of room. You don't need to go more than ten meters per attempt. Repeat five times.

9. Alternate thirty to sixty seconds of running with sixty seconds of walking for a total of ten minutes, running through the frame questions of the mind-body stride drill and giving special focus to your running Pose and change of support. How do your shoulders feel lifting to unload body weight? Are you perceptive of counterbalancing with your arms and keeping your trunk upright, maintaining the S shape of your support leg and body?

10. For your strength routine, increase to twelve reps of each exercise.

11. Complete the post-session review in your running journal, recording your observations and feelings of body weight placement and Pose position with each landing. Reframe any frustrations you contended with. Did the heel of your support foot come off the ground as you fell forward? Could you feel you body falling forward from one running Pose to the next? Could you feel the position of your airborne foot? Was it making the number 4? What are your goals for your next training session?

LESSON EIGHT

Falling Frame Revisited

In this lesson you'll learn how speed is a consequence of your falling angle as opposed to the muscular efforts of pushing off and driving the knee forward. The greater the angle of falling, the faster you will run.

The photos below show runners moving at three different speeds: a jog, a run, and a sprint. These frames illustrate that speed is directly related to falling angle.

When I want to calculate a runner's falling angle, I isolate the fall frame and draw a vertex point where the ball of the foot touches the ground. From this point I draw a vertical line perpendicular to the ground and a slanted line that connects the vertex point to the center of the runner's hip.

Usain Bolt is the fastest guy in the world, and not by coincidence he has the

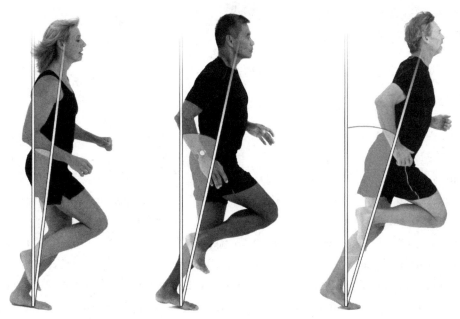

The greater the angle of falling, the faster the run

most extreme angle of falling. At top speed his angle is 21.4 degrees. At 22.5 degrees the physical laws of gravity take over and it is impossible to recover and land in the running Pose. Even Usain Bolt would stumble. Running at 21.4 degrees is daredevil stuff.

Falling angle also dictates how high the nonsupport foot is off the ground—a measure referred to as magnitude. The greater the fall angle, the closer your heel is to your butt and the faster you will be running. When you sprint, your angle of falling is at its greatest and your nonsupport leg is at its highest. By comparison, in a jog, your angle of falling is less extreme, and the magnitude of your foot is low.

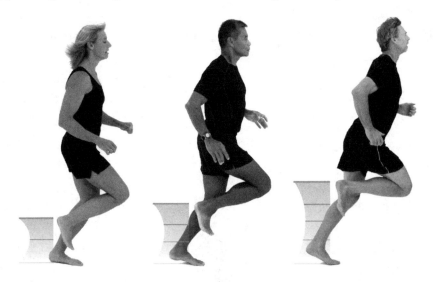

The greater the fall angle, the faster you run, and the higher you pull your leg

TECHNIQUE: FALL LIKE A RUNNER

Here's where it gets a little tricky. In Lesson Three you were taught to have your whole body fall as one piece. The goal of that lesson was to increase your perception of falling, but that's not the optimal way to fall when you run. True fall angle is measured from the support foot to the hip—meaning you should fall primarily from the waist down. Moreover, falling has a beginning and an end within the sequence of your stride. To get you comfortable with the idea of falling, I've implied that running is an act of constantly falling. But this isn't exactly the case. In truth, falling should start when the heel of the support foot moves off the ground, and it should end when the foot of your swing leg passes your support leg.

FOCUS PREPARATION

I look at the depictions of runners on the ancient Greek vases and their upright posture. I look at Michael Johnson's upright torso. That is my goal for the day. Keep my torso vertical. When I run I have to remember I fall from my hips, not full body falling like the early drills. The goal of those drills was to develop a perception of falling in my body, not the way I actually fall when I run. Technique intentions before today's run:

- Catch my body with my forefoot under my hip, which is Pose.
- Pull into Pose.

FALLING DRILLS REVISITED

The goal of this lesson's drills is to refine the falling phase of your stride.

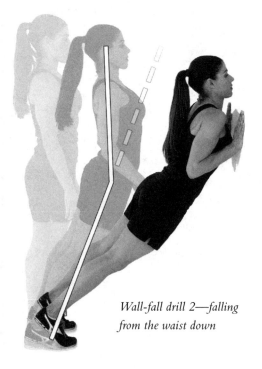

Wall-Fall Drill 2—Falling from the Waist Down

1. Get in your springiness position.

2. Prepare to fearlessly fall.

3. Fall forward into the wall, leading with your hips and keeping your upper body vertical.

4. Catch yourself with your hands.

Wall-fall drill 2—falling from the waist down

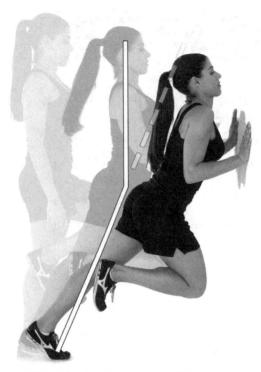

Wall-fall in the Pose position drill 2—falling from the waist down

Wall-Fall in Pose Position Drill 2—Falling from the Waist Down

1. Assume the running Pose.

2. Prepare to fall.

3. Fall, keeping your upper body vertical as your hips move forward over your support foot.

4. Catch yourself with your hands.

5. Repeat with other leg as your support leg.

Timber Drill 2—Falling from the Waist Down

1. Get in the running Pose.

2. Fall forward out of Pose, keeping your upper body vertical as your hips move forward over your support foot.

3. Fall until you are forced to catch yourself with your nonsupport leg, landing in the running Pose. Be fearless.

4. Feel your heel kiss the floor and then rise again as your body weight centers on the ball of your foot and your hips are stable. They should not continue moving forward.

5. Repeat with other leg as your support leg.

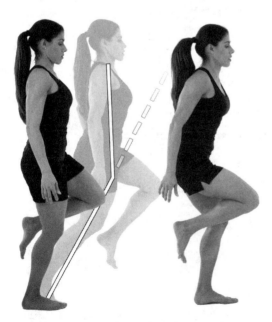

Timber drill 2—falling from the waist down

Falling Forward and Transition to a Run Drill

This is an elaboration on the change of support forward motion drill of the previous lesson; the timing and position of your falling phase are added to the mix of techniques you must master in the course of your stride.

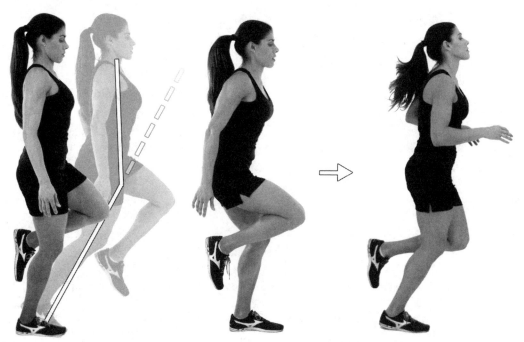

Falling forward and transition to a run drill

1. Get in the running Pose on your left leg, with the ankle of the swing leg at knee level.

2. Prepare to fearlessly fall.

3. Fall forward out of Pose, leading with your hips and keeping your upper body vertical.

4. When the foot of your swing leg passes your support leg, lift your shoulders to help unload body weight as you pull your left leg up under your hip, making sure your legs resemble the number 4 in profile.

5. Land on your right forefoot, letting your heel kiss the floor and then rise again as your muscle-tendon elasticity system stretches and recoils for release. Your hip should be directly above your support foot and your right leg should be bent slightly to form an S shape with your body.

6. As soon as you register your full body weight on the ball of your right foot, fall forward again—fearlessly!—keeping your upper body erect as your hips move forward past the ball of your right foot.

7. Repeat the sequence until you are back on the support foot you started with. This equals one stride.

8. Complete three strides in one continuous motion, moving forward for a total of six falls. Work on making the change of support fluid and precise, keeping your upper body erect and your arms loose as counterbalance to your legs.

9. Transition into a natural run for ten to twenty meters. Try to re-create the same angle of falling as you break into a run.

WORKOUT

1. Complete the focus preparation segment of your running journal.

2. Complete all three body weight perception drills—springiness position, running in place, and the running Pose.

3. Do the Pose hold drill for twenty seconds on each leg, for a set of three.

4. Complete five reps of wall-fall drill 2 from the springiness position, and five reps on each leg from the running Pose. Focus on falling from your lower body, keeping your upper body vertical.

5. Do three timber drills, two reps on each support leg. Raise your nonsupport foot to different levels in relation to your support foot: ankle, midcalf, knee.

6. Complete ten change of support drill reps, resting thirty seconds between each.

7. Complete ten to twenty reps of the base jump forward motion drill, rest for thirty to sixty seconds, and repeat for a total of three sets.

8. Engage in the falling forward motion drill, stringing together as many strides as you can, until you experience a breakdown in technique or you run out of room. You don't need to go more than ten meters per attempt. Repeat five times.

9. Alternate thirty to sixty seconds of running with sixty seconds of walking for a total of ten minutes, running through the frame questions of the mind-body stride drill and giving special focus to your falling frame. Are you keeping your upper body vertical as you fall forward from the waist down? Does your fall begin as soon as you feel your full body weight on the ball of your support foot and end when your swing foot passes your support knee?

10. For your strength routine, do twelve reps of each exercise.

11. Complete the post-session review in your running journal, recording your observations and feelings of falling from the waist down at the correct moments in each stride. Reframe any frustrations you contended with. How does it feel to fall from hips down? Can you sense a connection between keeping your upper body vertical and having your foot land under your hip? Can you feel the different degrees of falling as you increase and decrease your speed? What are your goals for your next training session?

LESSON NINE

Pulling Frame Revisited

You guessed it. In this lesson the pulling drills will get more dynamic, and you will zero in on the timing of the pull. I hope that I've convinced you already that efficiency and precision in changing support are *not* achieved by pushing off the ground and ankle extension. Efficiency and precision in changing support come through pulling and unloading weight.

TECHNIQUE

Let's take a look at the pull phase in more detail, zeroing in on its timing. Ideally, pulling begins when falling ends—as soon as the foot of the swing leg passes the support leg. Even elite runners don't nail this every time. The habit to catch yourself and land is so strong that it overcomes the desire you will cultivate in this lesson.

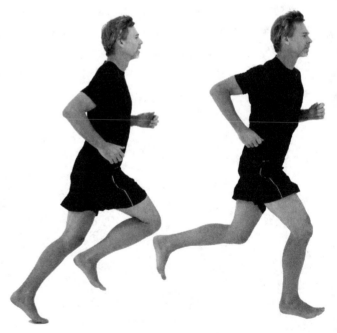

Moving past the threshold to pull

PULLING DRILLS REVISITED

These drills will force you to use your hamstring muscles to pull your foot from the ground directly under your hip, launching you into the flight phase, where both your feet are off the ground.

Foot Tapping and Transition to a Run Drill

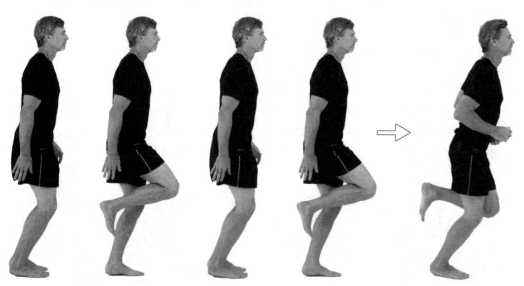

Foot tapping and transition to a run drill

1. Start in the running Pose on your left foot.

2. Focus on tapping the ball of your right foot, under your hip, then using the hamstring to pull your right foot from the ground back and up under your hip. The left foot will remain on the ground throughout the drill.

3. From the running Pose, let your right foot drop toward the ground and land on the forefoot under your hip is a quick tapping motion.

4. Allow your right heel to drop lightly to kiss the ground.

5. Use your right hamstring to quickly pull the right foot back up under your hip, shrugging your shoulders slightly to unload weight. Your right quad should stay relaxed and your right ankle should be lifted in a straight vertical line.

6. Repeat the sequence quickly, keeping ground contact time with your right foot to a minimum—the rhythm of pulling and landing should be fast up, slow down, while your left foot supports your body weight throughout.

7. As drill reps increase in speed, allow your left support leg to do a little hop in place with each lift of the right foot as you shrug your shoulders to unload weight. Remember to keep your knees bent and to land on the ball of your right foot every time.

8. Switch the support leg and repeat.

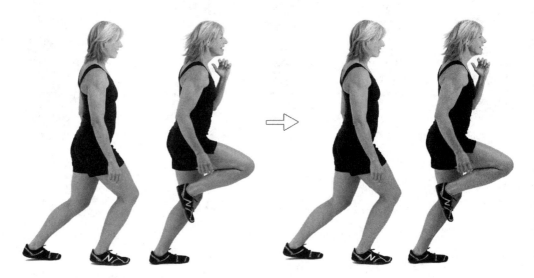

Front lunge with forward movement drill

Front Lunge with Forward Movement Drill

1. Using the above drill as a foundation, from the running Pose let the ball of your right foot drop to the ground and land under your hip, followed by a kiss of your right heel on the ground.

2. Shrugging your shoulders slightly to unload weight, quickly pull the right foot back up under your hip, using your hamstring and keeping your quad relaxed. As before, your right ankle should be lifted in a straight vertical line.

3. Fall forward, moving your hips over your point of support—the ball of your left foot.

4. Let your right foot drop toward the ground and land on the forefoot under your hip, while your left leg relaxes, allowing your left foot to quickly slide forward under the hip to serve as the support leg once more.

5. Repeat the sequence quickly, keeping ground contact time with your right foot to a minimum.

6. As drill reps increase in speed, allow your left support leg to do a little skip forward with each lift of the right foot as you shrug your shoulders to unload weight. Remember to keep your knees bent and to land on the ball of your right foot every time.

7. Switch the support leg and repeat.

WORKOUT

1. Complete the focus preparation segment of your running journal.

2. Complete all three body weight perception drills—springiness position, running in place, and the running Pose.

3. Do the Pose hold drill for twenty seconds on each leg, for a set of three.

5. Complete three reps of the wall-fall drill from the springiness position, and three reps on each leg from the the running Pose, moving farther away from the wall to challenge yourself.

6. Complete three timber drill reps on each support leg from the Pose position, raising your nonsupport foot to different levels in relation to your support foot: ankle, midcalf, knee.

7. Complete ten foot tap drill reps on each support leg, resting ten to fifteen seconds in between. Repeat for three sets on each leg.

8. Complete ten change of support drill reps, resting thirty seconds between each.

9. Complete ten to twenty reps of the base jump forward motion drill, rest for thirty to sixty seconds, and repeat for a total of two sets.

10. Engage in the change of support forward motion drill, stringing together as many strides as you can, until you experience a breakdown in technique or you run out of room. You don't need to go more than ten meters per attempt. Repeat five times.

11. Complete ten front lunge forward motion drill reps on each support leg, resting ten to fifteen seconds in between. Repeat for three sets on each leg.

12. Alternate thirty to sixty seconds of running with sixty seconds of walking for a total of ten minutes, running through the frame questions of the mind-body stride drill and placing special focus on your pulling frame. Are you keeping your quads relaxed with each pull, engaging your hamstring muscles to pull your ankle straight back and up from the ground directly beneath your hip? Are you launching into the flight phase as soon as your swing foot passes your support knee?

13. For your strength routine, do twelve reps of each exercise.

14. Complete the post-session review in your running journal, recording your observations and feelings of pulling with your hamstring at the correct moment in each stride. Reframe any frustrations you contended with. Did you keep contact time on the ground quick, just a tap? Could you perceive your hamstring doing the work? Were you pulling your ankle up in a straight vertical line? How did you do with the rhythm fast up and slow down? What are your goals for your next training session?

LESSON TEN

Putting It All Together Again

In this lesson you'll take your deeper knowledge and perception of running technique out for a twenty-minute run, integrating all that you've learned. This final lesson is also designed to be a running workout to take you seamlessly into the next phase of the program. But before you hit the road, I want to cover a biomechanical concept that has been at the root of all the lessons, from the maintenance of the S-shaped curve to the warnings against landing ahead of your center of mass. For optimum running, you must observe the body's natural patterns of *geometric restraint*. Don't worry. Your body is programmed to slow the movement of a joint down as it gets close to full extension. That's how you avoid injuries caused by hyperextension. So when you run you should never try to fully extend your legs. You should always pull your foot straight up under your hip, instead of kicking it way back behind you. You should always keep your knee slightly bent in the running Pose. This governing concept of geometric restraint allows you take advantage of the muscle-tendon elasticity that is movement's best friend.

TECHNIQUE

The technique goal of Lesson Ten is simple: integrate Pose, fall, pull into a slightly longer run. This is an expansion of the mind-body stride drill you've completed in the past few lessons—instead of focusing on one frame, you'll be exercising your perception with equal focus on the whole package, both during your run and during moments of rest.

VISUALIZATION DRILL

1. Find a quiet moment in your day to devote four minutes to a daydream—before you go to bed, on the subway, during a break at work, right before you run.

2. Imagine yourself running in perfect form. Use all your senses to create the imaginary scene. Really see and feel yourself running in the perfect Pose form. The following guidelines are some points of focus.

- **See** yourself running— from a distance, your full body—with perfect technique.

- **Feel** yourself land on the balls of your feet in perfect balance in the running Pose.

- **Hear** the soft, quick touch of your foot making contact with the ground.

- **Feel** the free falling sensation as you move forward.

- **Sense** that precise moment when you pull and launch into the flight phase.

TECHNIQUE CHECKLIST

This is a master checklist of questions that you can keep coming back to—not just this week, but every time you feel like your proper technique might be breaking down. Think of it as the ultimate mind-body stride drill. If you're struggling with perceiving a frame in your body, stop running and do a drill for that frame, then move right back into your run.

1. How do I perceive my running Pose? Do I land on the ball of my foot? Do I sense pressure on the ball of my foot on my support leg? Do I have my swing foot under my hip during support? Am I relaxed? Is my foot landing directly under my hip? Do my knees stay slightly bent, maintaining muscle elasticity? Does my Pose magnitude match my speed?

2. How do I perceive falling? Do I feel tension in my ankle? Do I feel an effortless movement forward? Do I maintain the running Pose when falling? Am I really giving in to it? Do I have muscular tension? Am I braking with any part of my body? Am I being courageous in experimenting with increasing my fall angle?

3. **How do I perceive pulling?** Am I pulling my foot directly under my hip? Do I perceive when falling ends? Am I sensing the right moment to pull? Am I pulling with correct magnitude to match my speed?

FOOT STRIKE COMPARISON

The following graphic will give a good visual summary of the basic concepts we've covered. It also takes us back to the core idea of landing in the optimal position.

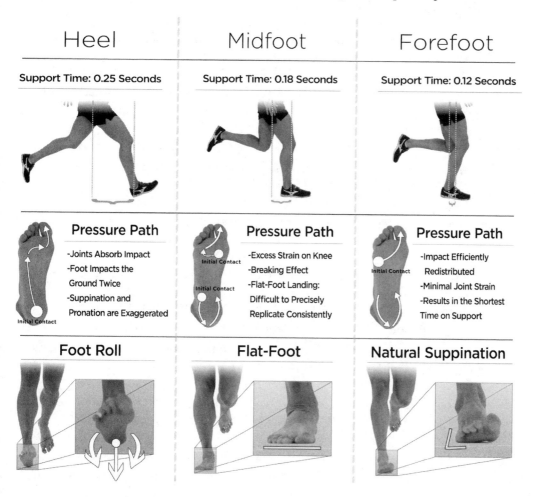

Foot strike comparison

WORKOUT

1. At least once a day starting today, set aside four minutes and complete a visualization drill.

2. In the focus preparation section of your journal, write down thoughts about the running technique you visualized, and how you will apply that vision to your run.

3. Complete all three body weight perception drills—springiness position, running in place, and the running Pose.

4. Do the Pose hold drill for twenty seconds on each leg, for a set of three.

5. Complete three reps of the wall-fall drill from the springiness position, and three reps on each leg from the running Pose, moving farther away from the wall to challenge yourself.

6. Complete three reps of timber drill number 2 on each support leg from the Pose position, raising your nonsupport foot to different levels in relation to your support foot: ankle, midcalf, knee.

7. Complete ten change of support drill reps, resting thirty seconds between each.

8. Complete ten to twenty reps of the base jump forward motion drill, rest for thirty to sixty seconds, and repeat for a total of two sets.

9. Engage in the change of support forward motion drill, stringing together as many strides as you can, until you experience a breakdown in technique or you run out of room. You don't need to go more than ten meters per attempt. Repeat five times.

10. Complete ten front lunge forward motion drill reps on each support leg, resting ten to fifteen seconds in between. Repeat for three sets on each leg.

11. Alternate thirty to sixty seconds of running with sixty seconds of walking for a total of twelve minutes, reviewing the questions of the technique checklist. If you're struggling with any of the frames, stop and do a drill for that frame, then move right back into your run.

12. Film yourself running. This should be at least your third digital capture. In the next chapter you'll learn how to analyze your form and apply your observations to the next phase of the Pose Method program.

13. For your strength routine, increase to fifteen reps of each exercise. This will be your strength regimen from now on.

14. Complete the post-session review in your running journal, recording your observations and feelings about every aspect of the technique checklist. Reframe any frustrations you contended with. How does it feel to integrate all the elements? What are the biggest challenges you face? What are some positive changes in running technique—mind and body? What are your goals as you move into the running circuit?

GRADUATION

Enjoying the Moment

Congratulations, you've completed your first ten lessons. Now you're going to put all this into practice in the running circuit phase of the program. Here are some pointers before you move forward, as well as a list of mistakes to avoid.

Be patient and go slow. Because you are learning a new movement pattern and using new muscles, you may experience some soreness. That's why quality is always more important than quantity. Doing the core exercises and jumps will help you make this transition. The most important thing is consistency. You need to commit to a minimum of three workouts a week.

Cadence, cadence, cadence. Focus on quick cadence and don't worry about extending your stride length. Your stride length is your stride length. It's like trying to make yourself taller. You can't do it. If you're doing everything right, stride length will take care of itself. That's good—it means you have one less thing to worry about.

Tune in to your beat. Focus on making your landing quiet. This means you're landing on the ball of your foot and taking advantage of muscle-tendon elasticity. If you're landing with a clomp, a slap, or a skid, this is not good. These are sounds of a less than optimal landing. Good running technique looks smooth and sounds quiet.

Fall forward from your hips over your point of support, keeping your upper body vertically aligned through your hip, shoulder, and head.

Land under your general center of mass. Land on the ball of your foot under your hip. This is your goal. If you miss the target a little, don't be too hard on yourself. Just avoid an active landing on your heel or ahead of your hips, creating a classic overstride. Landing under your hips helps you harness the power of forward momentum.

Film regularly. Make sure you film yourself on a consistent basis. This is the only way to analyze your mechanics. Once you get in the habit this will become an enjoyable part of the process.

CHECKLIST OF COMMON MISTAKES

- Overstriding
- Heel striking
- Active landing
- Pulling late
- Bending at the waist
- Resistance to falling
- Increased vertical oscillation (a lot of up and down movement)
- Excessive arm movement
- Overpulling
- Excessive noise on landing
- Scuffing and scratching on landing

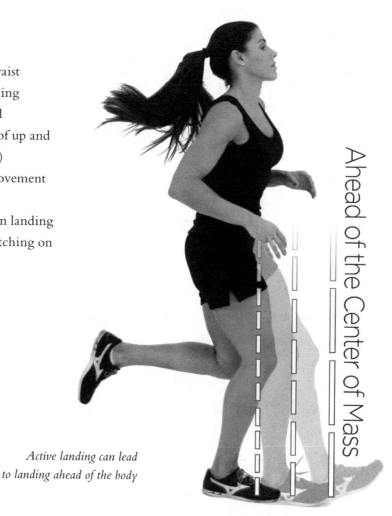

Active landing can lead to landing ahead of the body

Ahead of the Center of Mass

PART THREE

THE RUNNING CIRCUIT

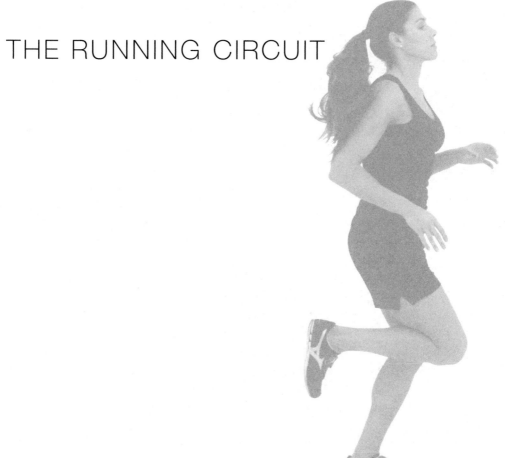

INTRODUCTION TO THE RUNNING CIRCUIT

Going to the Next Level

This nine-week transition period continues to be all about quality over quantity. The central part of the program is running intermixed with drills, like a circuit training workout for running—hence the "running circuit." Make sure you follow the regimen closely, including the close analysis of your video capture as set forth in the next chapter. As with the lessons, it may seem too easy in the beginning, but it quickly builds through a series of cumulative goals. Running and learning a new skill go deep into exercise physiology: musculoskeletal, physiological, neurological, and psychological. All these key elements of exercise physiology have their own timetable. It's like sautéing vegetables; fresh spinach cooks faster than potatoes. With your body you first make neurological adaptations, then your muscles get strong, but your tendons and ligaments (like the potato) need a little extra time to get strong. The different elements of the program make this efficient and safe.

BECOMING YOUR OWN COACH

Overcoming Challenges

Before you take another step, you must first learn how to analyze footage of your running stride. Video analysis is a crucial skill for this next phase of the program—the running circuit—since you'll be applying the drills directly to your running form, custom-tailoring your workouts to focus on your individual needs for improvement.

If you've been following my instructions, you should have at least three videos that capture your running form at various phases of the Pose Method program:

1. After you acquired your shoes and read the chapter on digital capture

2. At the beginning of Lesson One

3. At the end of Lesson Ten

Now is the time to pull these clips up on the computer screen—or better yet, the TV screen—and have a close look at them. Ideally, you should access them through a program that lets you view video frame by frame—a movie-editing program like iMovie or Movie Maker, for example. Otherwise, you'll want to upload the videos to YouTube, then paste the video links in a specialized viewing site like PauseHouse.com. There you'll be able to analyze, frame by frame, how closely your form matches the ideal Pose Method sequence. Here it is again and on page 109.

Now that you understand the concepts of Pose, you can start to analyze your running like a coach. Let's examine the qualities of the ideal form frame by frame.

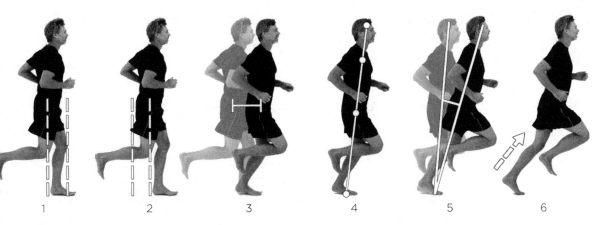

1. Initial contact. 2. Running Pose. 3. Heel lifts as the body begins falling. 4. Falling ends when the swing foot passes the support leg and trail leg pulls up. 5. Flight phase.

1. *Initial contact:* Foot lands in slight supination almost under the body. Trail leg is only slightly behind the body, minimizing time to Pose position.

2. *Trail leg distance:* The trail leg is slightly behind the body at initial contact.

3. *Pose position:* Upper body remains vertical as it passes through the Pose position.

4. *Falling begins:* As the body begins falling, the heel should lift off the ground.

5. *Falling ends:* The swing foot is past the support leg.

6. *Pull into flight:* Pulling the heel under the hip (the amount the swing foot passes the trail leg) initiates the flight phase.

Have a look at all three of your videos in slow motion, comparing your stride with the illustration above. Ideally, your form will show signs of improvement from one video to the next. Have another slow-motion look at the third video and jot down in your journal some general reflections on what you see:

- What are you doing right?
- What are you doing wrong?
- How can you correct mistakes?

Once you have a general idea of how to evaluate your stride, you'll be ready to break it down frame by frame, evaluating the three key positions: Am I in Pose? Am I falling? Am I pulling at the right time and correctly? The guidelines below will help you isolate deviations from form and enact a plan to correct those errors. Keep taking notes in your journal as you move through these frames.

VIDEO ANALYSIS: THE RUNNING POSE

The Pose stance, as you know, is your position of greatest balance. The better your Pose stance alignment, the greater your falling potential after you land. As you read through the following five steps, you will find the illustration on the previous page helpful as a reference. The illustration contains five figures, which I will refer to in the following breakdown.

1. *Setup:* Scan to a moment in the clip when you are in front of the camera and can see your stride clearly.

2. *Landing:* Stop at the frame in which your foot first makes landfall—with your body weight inclined toward the forefoot and your heel kissing the ground. Take a look at the position of your legs and support foot in relation to your body. (Figure 1) Ideally, your foot lands under your body, enabling your muscles and tendons to quickly absorb the load of your body weight and release the energy back into the movement. If you are landing with your foot and leg ahead of your hips (your general center of gravity), you're in a classic overstride, which will lock the ankle, knee, and hip joints, making these joints absorb the impact. Over time the weakest link fails, leading to injury, usually of the knee or the hip.

3. *Loading:* Click forward to the next video frame, when your foot starts to take on more body weight as you move toward the running Pose. (Figure 2) If your landing position was correct, this frame should depict a quick injection of load that doesn't jam the joints and doesn't ask the tendons to hold the load as if they were muscles. Tendons are designed to handle quick loads. Muscles are better at handling slow loads and stability chores.

4. *The running Pose:* Start counting frames. How many frames does it take you to get into Pose—with your body weight on the forefoot and your heel slightly off the ground? (Figure 2) At thirty frames per second, the standard to aim for in reaching the running Pose is one to two frames. If it takes four frames from first touch to Pose stance, then you are likely reaching out ahead of your body in a classic overstride.

5. *Pose position alignment:* Once you are in the running Pose, you need to evaluate if you are in vertical Pose alignment with your foot under your hip or if you are leaning forward with your swing foot trailing your body. (Figure 4) If you are in the running Pose falling forward—say, 5 degrees past vertical—then you have given up 5 degrees of your falling potential and are running slower than you could be with the same effort. (If you are more than 22.5 degrees past vertical, you are about to do a face plant.) Ideally, you are in the vertical Pose (Figure 3) before you start the fall phase (Figure 5). How many frames does it take for the heel of the support foot to rise off the ground to pull? If it takes you two frames to get into the running Pose and four frames to get out, you're pulling too late.

VIDEO ANALYSIS: FALLING

1. *Setup:* Scan to a moment in the clip when you are in front of the camera and can see your stride clearly.

2. *Running Pose:* Stop at the frame in which you are in your optimum Pose stance alignment. (Figure 2)

3. *Unloading:* Click forward to the frame in which the heel of your support leg rises off the ground—this is the beginning of falling, when the majority of your body weight will move off the ball of your foot toward your swing leg. (Figure 3)

4. *Falling:* Start counting frames. How many frames does it take for the heel of the support foot to rise to its maximum height off the ground—the last frame before you pull your foot off the ground? (Figure 4) The standard at thirty frames per second is one to two frames, so if it takes you four frames to fall out of the running Pose for the pull, you're pulling too late. The instant the swing leg passes the threshold of the knee of the support leg, you should be done falling and your support foot should be entering the pull phase.

5. *Falling alignment:* As you click through the falling frames, check your body position. You should be maintaining Pose alignment from the hips up. Many runners try to use the trunk to lean forward, thinking that bending at the waist increases their fall angle. But Newton's Third Law never sleeps—the action of bending from the waist has to be countered by the trailing leg, causing you to keep your support foot on the ground too long, unbalancing your whole system. Some of our coaches call this beginner error the K Position Error because the form resembles the letter "K."

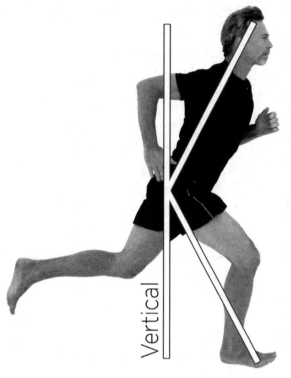

The K position error

Another seemingly obvious but common error is to not allow your body to fall at all. This means your heel is not leaving the ground and your upper body is rigid over your feet, effectively putting on the brakes. You're holding back out of fear of falling and fear of increasing your speed. In another few frames you'll be making the most common pulling error, which we'll examine in detail in the next section: the push off and knee drive to propel your body forward.

VIDEO ANALYSIS: PULLING

Pulling is the primary action of running, and the magic happens when you pull on time.

1. *Setup:* Scan to a moment in the clip when you are in front of the camera and can see your stride clearly.

2. *Change of support:* Stop at the frame where your swing foot passes your support leg, signaling the end of falling. (Figure 4)

3. *Flight phase:* Start counting frames. How many frames does it take for your support foot to leave the ground, initiating flight phase, when both feet are off the ground? (Figure 5) The answer should be zero. If your support foot is touching the ground after more than one frame, you are pulling too late.

4. *Pulling:* Continue counting frames. How many frames does it take for your pulling foot to lift directly under your hip into the running Pose while your other foot lands? The gold standard is, once again, one to two frames from flight phase launch to landing in the running Pose.

5. *Pulling position:* Rewind and view your pulling leg position frame by frame. Your foot should rise up directly under your hip, so that your pulling ankle is level with your opposite knee, making the shape of a number 4 with your lower body. (Figure 2) Watch for signs of over-pulling, in which you pull the foot too high toward your butt for the speed at which you're running. Also look for signs of attempting to push off. This overextends your joints and doesn't allow you to take advantage of your best friend: muscle-tendon elasticity. It also leads to the most common pulling error: pulling your foot behind your hip instead of directly under your hip. And finally, check for the ultimate error of the seventies: the knee drive, using the knee or thigh to pull the leg up.

Having analyzed thousands of participants in Pose running clinics, I've found that many people fully believe they are pulling their foot from the ground correctly until video analysis reveals the true story: They are not directly pulling their foot under their hips. Quite often this is the result of underdeveloped hamstrings. At certain speeds you can get away with this by falling late with a late pull, but at faster speeds this becomes a real problem. To achieve the perfect pull, you have to develop a mental image of pulling your foot from the ground under the hip and into the running Pose.

VIDEO ANALYSIS: YOUR UPPER BODY

Throughout the Pose Method sequence, your trunk must remain upright and be strong enough to provide support for your arms and legs to move freely, so your body can move forward efficiently. Always concentrate on the fact that the work is being done underneath the trunk, not by the trunk. Just as the chassis of a car is transported by the movement of the wheels and contributes nothing to its forward progress, the trunk of your body is just along for the ride and should do nothing to impede smooth progress down the road.

1. Starting with the frame you left off with in the pulling analysis, move frame by frame through the next stride sequence in your video, focusing on your upper body. Note in your journal any frames in which your torso is bending forward or backward—even if it's throughout your entire stride. Again, make sure your body is not making that special K shape.

2. Continue moving through the video, frame by frame, this time examining the movement of your arms. Remember that the main function of your arms is to provide a counterbalance to your legs, moving minimally, synchronized with your lower body to keep you moving forward with the greatest efficiency. Note whether your arms are moving side to side, or if they're overpumping (in which case you're probably engaged in a push off/knee-drive sequence that needs to be corrected).

CORRECTING YOUR ERRORS

Now that you've learned to examine your form with the ruthless objectivity of a coach, you know what corrective measures need to be taken. Below is a series of exercises to address the errors you discovered while analyzing your form on film. As you move forward into the running circuit phase of the Pose Method program, you'll want to incorporate the pertinent exercises into your movement preparation and strength routines.

Running Pose Stability: Holding the Pose Barefoot

Place a small object on the ground, such as a book or, for an extreme challenge, a medicine ball. Stand on the object in the running Pose; have only the ball of your foot on the object for support. Your heel hangs over the edge. You can also do this on a stair. The exercise heightens your sensitivity to your body weight's location and strengthens stability muscles.

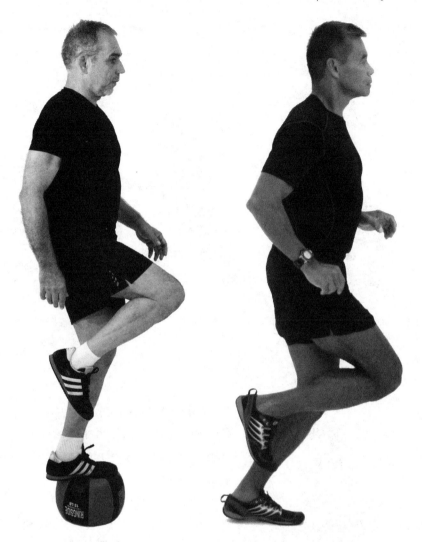

Running Pose stability   *Running Pose alignment*

Running Pose Alignment: Correcting the Vertical Line

Either take a picture of yourself or have a friend take a photo of you standing in the running Pose. Now compare this picture with the Pose standard. Make any necessary corrections by moving your shoulders, hips, knees, arms, or head in alignment with your support foot. If you can't get a photo taken, check yourself in a mirror or have a partner move you into the proper position. Once you see the error, your perception increases and it's easier to correct.

Falling Alignment: Correcting Bending at the Waist

Overexaggerate the bend. Bend over at a comical angle, then bring your spine and shoulders into alignment as you straighten back up.

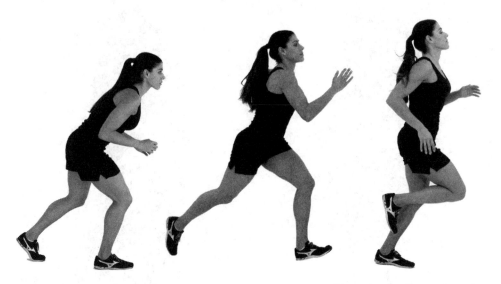

Correcting bending at the waist

Falling Alignment: Correcting the K Position

Hop on two legs in your springiness position. This prevents bending at the waist. You can do the same correction exercise by hopping on one leg in the running Pose. This is, obviously, more advanced, so master the two-leg hop first.

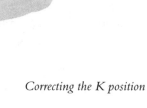

Correcting the K position

Pulling Speed: Correcting the Late Pull

What if your frame count of getting in and out of the running Pose is equal: three frames to get in and three frames to get out of Pose, or four to get in and four to get out. This would mean you don't have an imbalance, so what's happening? You're doing everything too slowly and you need to do it all faster. You need to increase strength and elasticity. The best exercise for this is jumping rope. It's good to jump barefoot, but regardless of your footwear, the key thing is perception. As you jump, focus on landing on the balls of your feet, so you feel the natural spring action of your feet. The more you jump rope, the faster your pull will become.

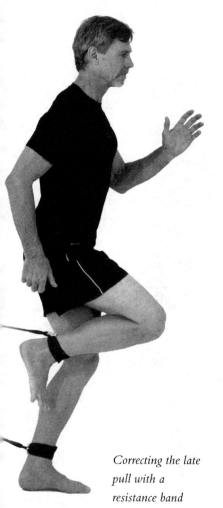

Correcting the late pull with a resistance band

Pulling Position: Correcting the Late Pull

Strong hamstrings are essential in developing the action of pulling. You can use numerous strength and conditioning exercises with ankle weights, rubber bands, weight machines, or your partner's resistance. You want to simultaneously develop your perception of pulling your foot while strengthening the muscles that do the work of the pull: your hamstrings. Many recreational runners have poorly developed hamstrings and a very low to nonexistent perception of what it feels like to pull the feet from the ground.

1. Standing with your feet hip–width apart, attach a cable or resistance band to one ankle with the anchor or resistance point behind your body.

2. Assume springiness position.

3. Keeping your torso upright, bring your heel toward your buttock without moving your thigh as you exhale—keep the thigh of your working leg even with your support leg and don't arch your back.

4. Inhale as you return to the starting position and repeat.

5. Switch legs, keeping your core activated for the entire set.

Here's a variation with ankle weights.

1. Securing it snugly, wrap the weight around your right ankle.

2. Place both hands against a wall or a chair for support.

3. Keeping your torso upright and your core engaged, lift your right knee off the floor as you exhale, simultaneously curling your foot toward your butt.

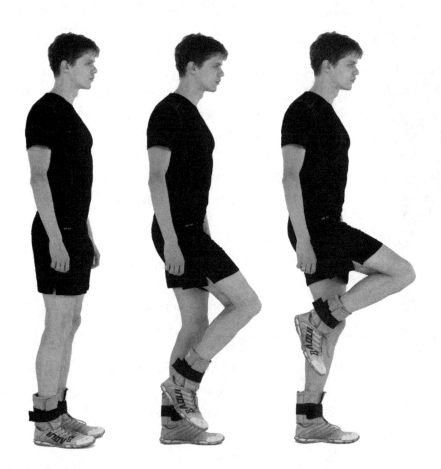

Correcting the late pull with ankle weights

4. Pause for a count and slowly lower your leg back to the floor as you inhale.

5. Repeat.

6. Switch legs, keeping your core activated for the entire set.

7. Reduce your support to one hand, eventually doing the move with no support, as illustrated.

Change of Support: Correcting the Slow Launch into Flight Phase

1. Start in the running Pose on your left leg with ankle weights secure on both legs. For an added challenge, stand on a deflated ball, as illustrated.

2. Pull your left leg under your hip. This foot has to leave the ground before the other foot drops.

3. Let your right foot naturally drop to the ground with no muscular effort.

4. Land on the ball of your right foot in perfect Pose position.

5. Repeat with your right leg, pulling it under your hip, shifting your weight, and landing on your right leg in perfect Pose.

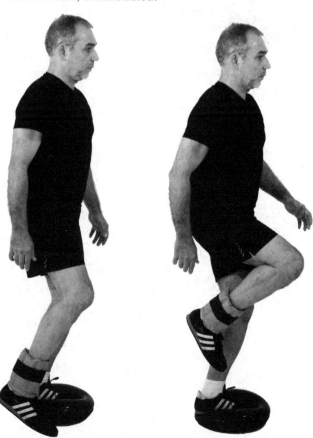

Correcting ankle stability with ankle weights

Upper Body: Correcting the Unstable Torso

One of the simplest ways to check for a stable trunk is to run with your arms extended in front of you at shoulder level, palms facing each other and the fingers interlaced.

TAKING YOUR COACHING TACTICS TO THE NEXT LEVEL

You've been training and thinking like an elite athlete (or a passionate runner deep into the process of improvement, depending on your mind-set). You've been filming and analyzing your running technique and gaining higher levels of perception, then you have been putting this knowledge to work when you run, creating a productive loop of perception and practice. Now, you also have a set of corrective tools to take your Pose Method training to the next level. As you move through the running circuit set forth in the next chapter, you'll be filming yourself and analyzing your form every three weeks at minimum. Since correcting some errors can allow other errors to creep in, you'll need to pay close attention to every moment of your stride, applying these corrective measures as needed.

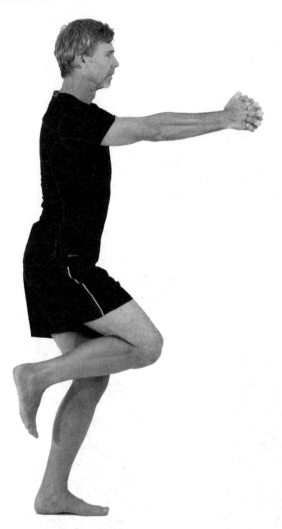

Correcting the unstable torso

THE RUNNING CIRCUIT

Making the Transition

The next stage of the program builds on the ten lessons of the last section, as well as the film analysis and corrective exercises you mastered in the previous chapter. It consists of a nine-week calendar of workouts to help you transition into running more distance in proper Pose Method—whether that be a 5K or an ultramarathon. Though it occupies the shortest chapter of the book, the running circuit will be the longest part of the program for you. Don't rush it.

Which brings us to an upgrade on your strengthening regimen.

STRENGTH ROUTINE UPGRADE

Remember back in Part One, when I warned that more challenging variations on your strength routine would be introduced later on? Well, here we are. If you've been vigilant about doing these exercises throughout the lessons, you should be ready for level two of the strength routine. When you get to this part of the workout in the running circuit, apply these variations.

Face-Up Hip Dips with One Leg Extended

1. Sit on the floor with your hands behind you and directly under your shoulders (palms down, fingers pointing away from your feet) and with your legs extended in front of you.

2. Raise and extend your left leg about eighteen inches off the floor.

3. Raise your hips up as high as you can, while supporting your body weight on your hands and right heel.

4. Return to the starting position and repeat for a set of ten.

5. Repeat with the other leg.

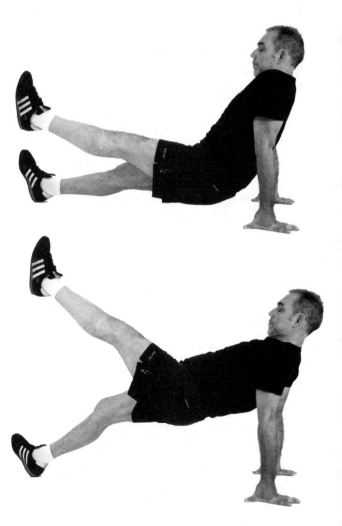

Face-up hip dips with one leg extended

Face-Down Hip Dips with One Leg Extended

1. Assume a push-up position, with a sagged hip and your hands directly under your shoulders, arms extended, hips level with your body, and toes tucked, then raise your right leg off the floor approximately six inches.

2. Move the hips straight up in the air, making an upside-down V, similar to yoga's downward dog position, while extending your right leg so it is level with your hip (a straight line from your right ankle to your right ear). You are now using only one leg for support. Keep your hips level; don't let them swivel.

3. Return to starting position and repeat for a set of ten.

Face-down hip dips with one leg extended

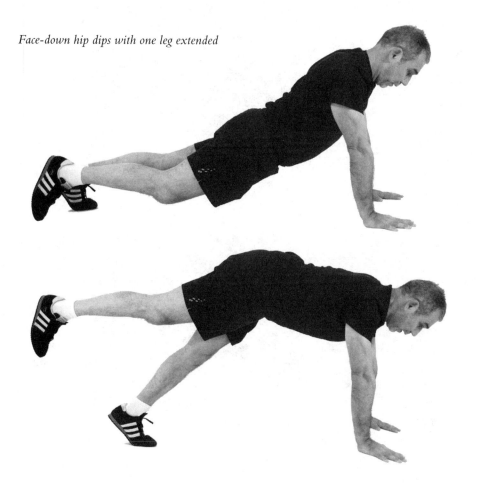

Side Hip Dips with One Leg Extended

1. Get in a side plank position with your right arm extended and your right hand under your shoulder supporting your torso, hips resting on the ground.

2. Raise your left leg, bringing it about twelve inches directly above your right leg.

3. Raise your hip straight up as high as you can.

4. Lower your hip back to the starting position and repeat for a set of ten.

5. Switch sides and do ten more reps.

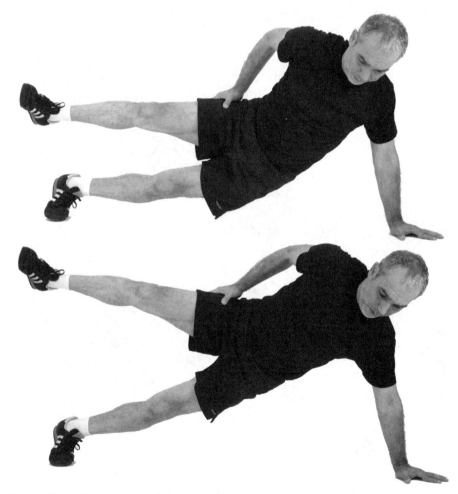

Side hip dips with one leg extended

Body Weight Squat with Heels Raised

1. Stand with your feet slightly wider than shoulder-width apart, hands extended straight ahead at shoulder level.

2. Shift your weight forward so that the balls of your feet are supporting all of your body weight.

3. Lower your hips, sitting down and back as far as you can into a squatting position, keeping your body weight on the balls of your feet.

4. Return to the starting position and repeat for a set of ten.

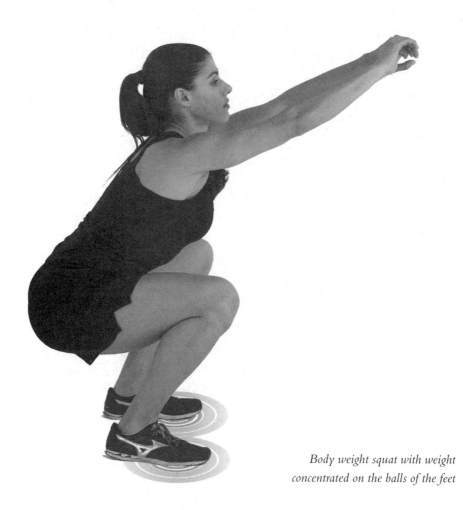

*Body weight squat with weight
concentrated on the balls of the feet*

THE RUNNING CIRCUIT DESIGN

Put it all together, and you have a plan for the next nine weeks. The running circuit consists of four rounds of drills, each of which includes a timed interval of running. You will be expected to complete a session three times a week, taking a day off between workouts (with a two-day break each week). If you miss a workout, don't move on to next week's plan until you've completed the current plan three times in one week.

The workouts are designed for you to run at a pace that is comfortable for your fitness level—always remember that you are mastering a new technique, not going after a personal record. The purpose of the running segment is not to build speed, but to integrate the drills gradually into your natural run with the ultimate goal of putting them all together. Don't try to overthink this. Just give yourself a simple cue phrase like "bring it all together" or "integrate," and let the wisdom of your body take over.

You will continue to preface every workout with a pre-session focus section in your journal and the movement preparation drills you've been completing from the start, and you will end each workout with the strength routine just like you did for your lessons. So this is your agenda three times a week:

1. Focus preparation in your journal

2. Movement preparation routine

3. Running circuit set forth in the table below

4. Strength routine—fifteen reps per exercise, upgraded to level two

5. Post-session review in your journal

Finally, remember to complete a video capture at the end of weeks three, six, and nine—marked with an asterisk on the schedule below.

THE NINE-WEEK SCHEDULE

Week	Round One	Round Two	Round Three	Round Four
1	Pose hold drill (p. 93), thirty seconds on each leg, followed by a three-minute run with focus on the running Pose.	Timber drill 2 (p. 126), three times on each leg, followed by a three-minute run with focus on falling.	Change of support drill (p. 105) three times on each leg, followed by a three-minute run with focus on pulling.	Drill of choice, followed by three-minute run with focus on integrating all the day's drill work into your run.
2	Pose hold drill (p. 93), thirty seconds on each leg, followed by a four-minute run with focus on the running Pose.	Timber drill 2 (p. 126), three times on each leg, followed by a four-minute run with focus on falling.	Change of support drill (p. 105), three times on each leg, followed by a four-minute run with focus on pulling.	Drill of choice, one minute total, followed by four-minute run with focus on integrating all the day's drill work into your run.
3*	Pose hold drill (p. 93), thirty seconds on each leg, followed by a five-minute run with focus on the running Pose.	Timber drill 2 (p. 126), three times on each leg, followed by a five-minute run with focus on falling.	Change of support drill (p. 105), three times on each leg, followed by a five-minute run with focus on pulling.	Drill of choice, one minute total, followed by five-minute run with focus on integrating all the day's drill work into your run.
4	Foot tap drill (p. 131), three times on each leg, building toward front lunge forward motion drill (p. 132) for ten meters straight into a six-minute run with focus on the running Pose and pulling.	Timber drill 2 (p. 126), three times on each leg, building toward falling forward motion drill (p. 127) for ten meters straight into a six-minute run with focus on falling.	Change of support drill (p. 105), three times on each leg, building toward change of support forward motion drill, (p. 120) for ten meters straight into a six-minute run with focus on pulling.	Drill of choice, followed by a six-minute run with focus on integrating all the day's drill work into your run.
5	Foot tap drill (p. 131), three times on each leg, building toward front lunge forward motion drill (p. 132) for ten meters straight into a six-minute run with focus on the running Pose and pulling.	Timber drill 2 (p. 126), three times on each leg, building toward falling forward motion drill (p. 127) for ten meters straight into a six-minute run with focus on falling.	Change of support drill (p. 105), three times on each leg, building toward change of support forward motion drill (p. 120) for ten meters straight into a six-minute run with focus on pulling.	Drill of choice, followed by a six-minute run with focus on integrating all the day's drill work into your run.

Week	Round One	Round Two	Round Three	Round Four
6*	Foot tap drill (p. 131), three times on each leg, building toward front lunge forward motion drill (p. 132) for ten meters straight into a six-minute run with focus on the running Pose and pulling.	Timber drill 2 (p. 126), three times on each leg, building toward falling forward motion drill (p. 127) for ten meters straight into a six-minute run with focus on falling.	Change of support drill, (p. 105) three times on each leg, building toward change of support forward motion drill (p. 120) for ten meters straight into a six-minute run with focus on pulling.	Drill of choice, followed by a six-minute run with focus on integrating all the day's drill work into your run.
7	Change of support drill, (p. 105) three times on each leg, building toward change of support forward motion drill (p. 120) for ten meters straight into a six-minute run with focus on pulling.	Timber drill 2 (p. 126), three times on each leg, building toward falling forward motion drill (p. 127) for ten meters straight into a seven-minute run with focus on falling.	Foot tap drill (p. 131), three times on each leg, building toward front lunge forward motion drill (p. 132) for ten meters straight into a seven-minute run with focus on the running Pose and pulling.	Drill of choice, followed by a six-minute run with focus on integrating all the day's drill work into your run.
8	Change of support drill, (p. 105) three times on each leg, building toward change of support forward motion drill (p. 120) for ten meters straight into a six-minute run with focus on pulling.	Timber drill 2 (p. 126), three times on each leg, building toward falling forward motion drill (p. 127) for ten meters straight into a seven-minute run with focus on falling.	Foot tap drill (p. 131), three times on each leg, building toward front lunge forward motion drill (p. 132) for ten meters straight into a seven-minute run with focus on the running Pose and pulling.	Drill of choice, followed by a six-minute run with focus on integrating all the day's drill work into your run.
9	Change of support drill, (p. 105) three times on each leg, building toward change of support forward motion drill (p. 120) for ten meters straight into a six-minute run with focus on pulling.	Timber drill 2 (p. 126), three times on each leg, building toward falling forward motion drill (p. 127) for ten meters straight into an eight-minute run with focus on falling.	Foot tap drill (p. 131), three times on each leg, building toward front lunge forward motion drill (p. 132) for ten meters straight into a seven-minute run with focus on the running Pose and pulling.	Drill of choice, followed by a six-minute run with focus on integrating all the day's drill work into your run.
*Video Capture				

TROUBLESHOOTING

To troubleshoot each phase—Pose, fall, pull—you will need to isolate your problem areas, apply corrective strategies, then integrate the correction(s) back into your stride. In the last chapter, "Becoming Your Own Coach," we gave you important skills and techniques for analyzing your running video, along with correction strategies. Mastering that process and having a troubleshooter's mind-set will be keys to your success.

As you work your way through the running circuit, you will need to consciously keep building your powers of mental concentration. In Pose, this is closely connected to perception. You need to deeply tune in to what is happening in your body when you run. This doesn't always mean a laser focus; more often it is a relaxed, whole-body attentiveness. It is about moment-to-moment awareness and not letting your mind wander into distraction about work, dinner, or a fight you just had with your significant other. An important tool in this process is your running journal.

The following guide will give you drills and exercises for each phase of Pose and examples of journal entries. If you're struggling with one of the phases, give extra emphasis to the prescribed drills and exercise, working up to three sets, resting a minute between sets. Spending a little extra time with prescribed drills and putting your thoughts on paper will help you conquer the challenges of learning a new technique.

TROUBLESHOOT YOUR LANDING

Your two biggest challenges are likely to be landing on your forefoot and landing with your foot under your hip. You will need to continually reinforce this.

CONSISTENTLY HITTING MY SWEET SPOT

Each time I land, I want to hit my forefoot, my sweet spot. When I hit my sweet spot, running feels effortless and I don't feel any wear and tear on my body. I'm struggling to hit it consistently on each landing. I still have a tendency to fade into a heel strike. It's easy to hit my sweet spot when I run in place. I can't even imagine running in place with a heel strike. It hurts just to think about it. But it becomes a challenge to land bull's-eye on my sweet spot when I go into motion. I need to take the mechanics of running in place into motion. I'm going to run in place for about ten to twenty seconds before I start my run.

Prescription

The following drills and exercise are helpful in getting you in touch with your sweet spot.

- Drill: body perception exercise
- Drill: foot tap to jog drill
- Exercise: full body squat

A BAREFOOT EXPERIMENT

As an experiment, I went for a barefoot run on a patch of grass in the park. I went for just a short distance, about forty meters. The run was all about trying to get in touch with my sweet spot, my perfect landing. Running barefoot I noticed these differences as compared to when I wear shoes:

- My landing was softer.
- I landed on the ball of my foot.
- I landed with my foot pretty much under my hip.
- My upper body stayed more vertical.

- My mind totally stayed focused. It could have been out of fear or just that it was a new experience. My awareness was definitely on high alert. One of the hardest parts of Pose is staying mentally aware stride after stride and not zoning out, slipping back into my old running pattern.

TROUBLESHOOTING YOUR FALLING

Falling, although it sounds easy, is also a big challenge (but for a different reason), because it is about letting go, or doing less. It triggers a psychological fear you also have to overcome—that you will not be able to catch yourself each time, that you will stumble. You need to keep practicing your falling drills. For the basic drill, tune in to the perception of falling, then add forward motion, maintaining the heightened perception of falling into your sequence of strides.

FEAR OF LETTING GO

I'm struggling with falling. I'm still trying to control things too much, the tyranny of the old pattern. I have short sequences when I'm falling, then I lapse back into what I might call safe running. I'm landing with my foot out in front of my body, not underneath my hip. It seems like falling is a bit of a paradox; you have to let go and at the same time it is an act of will, at least when I'm trying to learn this new way of running.

Prescription

The following drills and exercise are helpful in getting you in touch with falling.

- Drill: timber drill
- Drill: falling forward motion to run drill
- Exercise: base jump with forward motion

FEAR OF LETTING GO

When I first heard about the forefoot strike, I thought it was something I actively went after, the same way I actively executed a heel strike. It was a revelation when Dr. Romanov explained that the forefoot strike is a consequence of falling, not something you actively do. I couldn't quite wrap my mind around that. So much of the new technique has all been about the forefoot strike versus the heel strike that it was hard for me not to actively try to forefoot strike. I thought it was going to be a simple substitution of one for the other. But it's not that simple. It's more like a complete overhaul. I have to let go and fall, catching myself on my forefoot, under my hip. I have to keep doing my fall drills to increase my falling perception.

TROUBLESHOOTING YOUR PULLING

Last but not least, you will face the challenge of pulling. Pulling is often the biggest hurdle to optimal running. It's easy to pull too late and to over-pull. Pulling is that instance when you actively pull the foot under your hip and launch into the flight phase. Since this is a muscular action it's important to build strength for this move. If you're really struggling with pulling and you consider body strength something you need to work on, then the first step is to increase your hamstring strength.

FEAR OF LETTING GO

When I run today, I want to feel myself hitting the running Pose as a dynamic instance in the support phase and focus more on pulling. I feel like I've trapped myself into thinking of the running Pose as more static than dynamic. This is making me pull late.

I want to indulge in pulling: feel my hamstring pull my foot toward my butt, feel the mechanics of the pull get released the microsecond my swing foot moves past the support leg, feel the right magnitude, how high I pull the leg toward my butt, exactly matching how fast I'm running. Trying to feel the connection between pull height and speed. Pulling lifts the body into the flight phase. When I run: I fall. I fly. I land.

Prescription

The following drills and exercise are helpful in getting you in touch with pulling.

- Drill: change of support drill
- Drill: change of support forward motion drill
- Exercise: heel touch jump

SETTING PRIORITIES AND CONFUSION

I need to prioritize. Here's a list of what I need to think about for my runs this week.

- Let go of forefoot striking as something I do, like the way I used to actively heel strike.
- Let my strike be a consequence of falling.
- Focus on pulling.
- Catch myself under my hip.
- Spend as little time as I can on support.

I need to remind myself: It's okay to be confused. It's okay to struggle. I've been running one way for a long time and that pattern is deeply ingrained. It's my default pattern, so I drift back to it. I'm also using muscles in a new way. Pose is hard because it is about letting go, using less effort, being more efficient. I feel more comfortable with effort. I feel like I'm working hard. The old Protestant work ethic. With Pose, I'm being asked to let go, to do less. This makes me feel guilty and I resist it.

LOVE THE PROCESS

Since everyone's challenge is unique, how you apply troubleshooting strategies will depend on your needs. Different challenges may arise in various phases of the running circuit. You will be in the process of isolating, correcting, and integrating. Ultimately the goal is integration. Even the best runners are always fine-tuning.

You will be tweaking and tuning your stride for the rest of your life. This is the great thing about the art and science of running and why so many people love it. It is an ongoing process of learning and improvement.

A final takeaway: An exercise that is useful to do before every workout is the visualization drill outlined on p. 136. You will get better and better at visualizing the more you practice it. It will have big payoffs if you do it consistently. Also, the Pose community and Web site give you a powerful troubleshooting resource.

TROUBLESHOOTING DRILLS

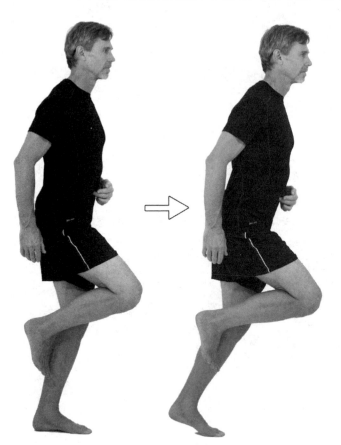

Belly button drill

Belly Button Drill

The purpose of this drill is to check if you are falling. You can do this test anytime during your run.

1. As you are running, lightly place your middle and index fingers on your belly button.

2. Fall into your finger with each stride.

3. If there's no pressure against your fingers, then you're not really falling. Focus on letting go and falling from your center with each stride.

Palm on Lower Back

The purpose of this drill is to check the position of your upper body. You can do this test at any time during your run.

1. As you are running, lightly place the palm of either hand on your lower back.

2. Try to sense if you are bending forward, trying to drive into your run. If you are, bring your torso to the correct upright position.

3. If you feel your lower back unnaturally arched, then bring your spine back to neutral (its natural curve).

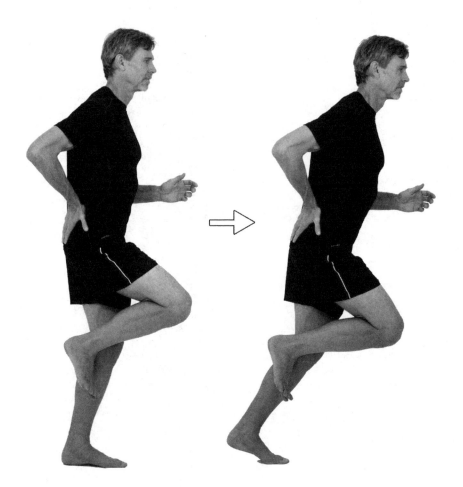

Palm on lower back drill

Hands Clasped in Front of Your Body

The purpose of this drill is to check on overstriding, late pulling, and leaning too far forward. You can do this test anytime you're running.

1. As you are running, extend your arms in front of you at shoulder level, clasping your hands together.

2. If your arms move from side to side, you're overstriding.

3. If your arms move up and down, you're pulling late.

4. If your hands are pointing down, you're bending forward.

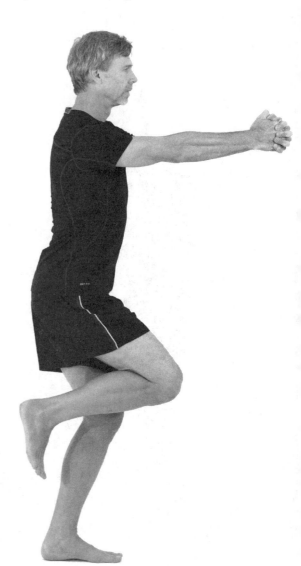

Hands clasped in front of your body

Hands Clasped Behind Your Body

The goal of this drill is to check if you're leaning too far forward and/or not landing with your foot under your hip. You can do this test anytime you're running.

1. As you are running, clasp your hands behind your back.

2. Is your upper body in an upright alignment or do you feel your torso bending forward?

3. Is your foot landing under your hips?

4. In either case, make the adjustments to an upright posture and/or focus on landing with your foot under your hip.

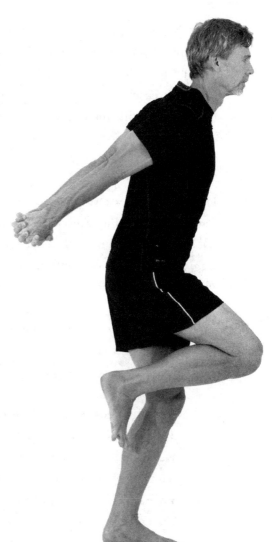

Hands clasped behind your body

RUNNING ON DIFFERENT SURFACES

All-Terrain Guide

While you'd be perfectly fine completing the entire running circuit part of the program on your regular running course, it's always a good idea—and a lot more fun—to shake things up with different surfaces and even reduced (or no) footwear.

This chapter will give you technique tips for running on treadmills, trails, and sand—up hills and down.

TREADMILLS

The treadmill is a tool to stay consistent in bad weather, during extremely cold winter days, or simply because it's more convenient. Sometimes circumstances make this the only practical choice. Treadmill running is not the same as road running, however, so some adjustments should be made. As always the goal is to run with optimal biomechanics and injury free.

- **Take off your shoes.** Running barefoot on the treadmill is a good way to get in touch with your sweet spot on the ball of your foot. If your gym prohibits barefoot running, do it in socks. Again use caution.
- **Set your treadmill inclination to 1 to 3 degrees.** This incline angle allows the body to fall forward as it does in road running.
- **Keep the body upright.** Don't grab the handles and bend forward. Stay in Pose alignment.
- **Focus on cadence.** In treadmill running this is primarily what changes when you increase or reduce the belt's speed. It is much easier to maintain high cadence while running on a treadmill. This increase in cadence can transfer to your road running.

TRAIL RUNNING

Trail running can be exhilarating—being off the beaten path, out in nature. You don't have to be in the woods or the mountains to do it. You can also trail run in city parks and greenbelts.

While road running provides a very uniform and stable surface, trails can change step by step. Running on an uneven surface filled with twists and turns can make it easier to twist an ankle or take a fall—in which case you'll want to turn to the next chapter on injuries and how to treat them.

But these hazards also have their advantages. When you trail run, your awareness and attention—and therefore perception—go up several notches and you tune in to what you are doing. The uneven surface and twists and turns lead to more well-rounded development of your muscles, ligaments, tendons, and joints. Teaching the lower body to land on the ground at a variety of angles and positions builds a more comprehensive strength foundation that will help keep you injury-free. Running in an unpredictable environment will develop an adaptive and adroit reactive system for running, training your neuromuscular system to be ready for a variety of situations. It is also great psychological training, preparing you to be ready for quick changes in running conditions without becoming unsettled or distracted.

If good trails are readily accessible, there is nothing wrong with making trail running the mainstay of your program, with relatively infrequent jaunts on traditional road surfaces. If you require a longer drive to get to your favorite trail, you might use it as a treat at the end of a training phase, a welcome psychological break from the normal day-to-day routine.

Here are some trail running tips:

- **Double your gaze.** Keep your gaze ahead to see what's coming up in the next ten to fifteen meters, while at the same time quickly checking the terrain directly in front of you for any danger signs in your next couple of strides.
- **Shorten your stride.** Because balance is essential, you need to shorten your stride so it is easier to land with your foot under your body and land on the ball of your foot. This is your optimal place of balance and it will help keep your foot from skidding and slipping.

- **Land lightly.** In trail running you need to be extraordinarily light on your feet and stay relaxed rather than tensing up.
- **Vary speed.** Recreational trail running is not about speed, but it offers a great opportunity to run at different paces. If the trail opens up to a nice smooth straightaway, take advantage and pick up your pace.

RUNNING ON SAND

Running on an uneven, soft, sandy beach may be one of the hardest workouts you'll ever do, while running on hard, packed sand will be a breeze. Either variety offers a multitude of benefits: It strengthens the muscles and ligaments, develops muscular balance in the legs, stabilizes your joints, develops aerobic capacity, hones your skills of interacting with the ground, and—perhaps most important—improves balanced muscular strength.

Additionally, running on sand makes it virtually impossible to overstride. If you are having problems breaking the habits of either pushing off with your foot on takeoff or landing on the heel and rolling through the midfoot to the toes, you'll find sand running a very effective tool in getting the feel of proper running technique. Digging your heel into the sand will cause you to quickly bog down. However, if you run with a light touch, landing on the ball of your foot with short strides, you won't penetrate nearly as far into the sand and you'll move along with more ease and speed.

Don't treat sand running as a workout in the conventional sense of time or distance, but instead as a contributor to your overall mastery of running technique and strength development. Soft sand automatically increases the intensity of the workout, like sprint work or running with a weight vest on. It increases the difficulty for both your muscles and your cardiovascular system. Expect your leg muscles to burn. Expect some serious huffing and puffing. Expect to be sore in your calves and quads, but realize that such soreness is an indication of ongoing strength development.

Here are some guidelines for the sand:

- **Start with short runs.** At the beginning, you should do runs mixed with walking intervals.

- **Technique first, not ego.** Run until you feel it impossible to maintain proper running technique; don't keep pushing it after your form breaks down.
- **Variety.** As your training program grows more rigorous, vary your approach to sand running, mixing in longer runs with tempo runs, medium intervals, sprints, and running on hard and soft sand.
- **Beware of the slope.** Beaches have somewhat severe slopes leading toward the water. Running only in one direction on these beaches can ultimately lead your body to subconsciously correct for this uneven terrain, which can in turn lead to debilitating injuries. Make sure to balance this out by running in both directions or moving farther away from the water where the slope is less severe.

UPHILL RUNNING

This may sound counterintuitive, but running uphill is easier than running downhill or even running on a flat surface, at least from a technique standpoint.

In uphill running, it's harder to make many of the mistakes that are easy to make when running on a flat surface (and even more tempting when running downhill). Uphill running causes you to reduce your stride. It's difficult to overstride, land on the heel, or push off when you are running uphill.

Here are guidelines for uphill running:

- Keep the same running Pose alignment while you run—don't bend forward.
- Run with shorter steps and a higher stride frequency.
- Keep your body weight on the balls of your feet.
- Keep your pull action short.
- Don't push off or straighten your legs.

DOWNHILL RUNNING

Downhill running is the most difficult to do with proper technique, because more gravity is available to you. So you need to adjust your technique to accommodate this increase in gravity. Instead of a focus on leaning forward, you need to concentrate on keeping your body straight, just above your point of support on the balls of your feet. You also need to be extra vigilant about landing with your feet under your hips. The tendency to overstride when running downhill can be irresistible. It is easy to start flying down a hill, but the consequences of increased impact on your legs out in front of your body will be extremely negative.

Your muscular efforts should also be reduced compared to running on a flat surface, and your pull of the foot from the ground should be minimal—just a little off the ground, with higher cadence than on the flat surface. By doing this you'll never lose control of your running pace. Here are some additional pointers:

- Keep your body aligned, with your weight above the point of support on the ball of your foot, as if you were running in place.
- Don't extend your feet out in front of your body. Land with your feet as closely under your hip as possible.
- Shorten your stride by focusing on pulling.
- Increase cadence.
- Keep your pull action short (just enough to break contact with the ground).

COMMON INJURIES

Prevention and Treatment

Common injuries in most cases originate from the cumulative effects of bad technique, which leads to overloading (more body weight at the wrong time and place) and misuse (making them do what they are not supposed to do) of support tissues. The first phase of an injury is the acute phase. During this phase you suffer pain and have to miss training days. As a result, you either self-medicate, just wait for the pain to subside, or get medical help. The good news: In all three scenarios, you usually get better. The bad news: The pain and injury frequently come back and you start the vicious cycle over again. Over time, the injury becomes chronic and something you just have to deal with.

The reason for this never-ending injury cycle is that you are treating the symptom, not the cause. You have to correct the technique flaw that is the cause of the injury. The approach in this chapter is to be a technique doctor. Injuries will be addressed by correcting the technique error, which is the root cause. The goal is to stop the injury cycle.

Your error will occur in one of the three Pose frames. By giving this frame special attention you will bring your deviation back to the standard. In this way your injuries can teach you hard but valuable lessons about your technique. The right diagnosis is key. Pain and injuries are almost always the result of how you land. Most of the problems are caused by overstriding (landing with your foot in front of your body) and bending at the waist. This puts your body in a vulnerable position. As the graphic below shows, most injuries happen during landing and more precisely during the first half of the support phase.

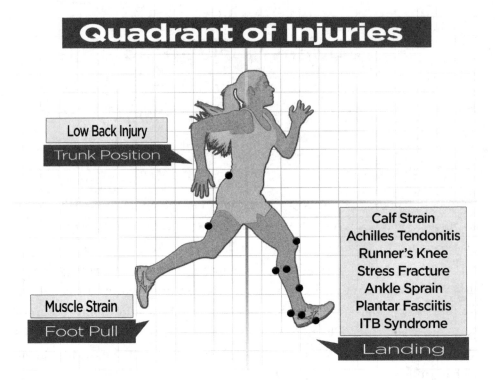

Quadrant of Injuries

Low Back Injury
Trunk Position

Muscle Strain
Foot Pull

Calf Strain
Achilles Tendonitis
Runner's Knee
Stress Fracture
Ankle Sprain
Plantar Fasciitis
ITB Syndrome

Landing

KNEE PAIN

The main cause of knee pain is landing ahead of your body (overstriding). This happens in two common ways:

- Landing ahead of body with a locked knee
- Landing ahead of your body with an overbent knee

Both of these variations put undue stress on the knee joint and the tendons, cartilage, and ligaments around the joint. The leg can't act like a spring when it lands ahead of the body or is locked. Thus, the joint absorbs the impact. The knee joint is not designed to bear extended weight and load. This is the job of the muscles.

Corrective

1. Fall forward and begin to run, focusing on pulling your foot under your hip and landing on the ball of your foot, feeling the natural spring action of the foot.

2. Run for twenty to thirty meters.

3. Repeat for three to five sets.

IT BAND PAIN

Since it is in the same quadrant as knee pain, it has a similar cause: landing ahead of your body. The main variation is what is defined as a wide landing with locked ankles and knees that do not allow forward progression of your hips.

This means you land outside the natural width of your hips (your feet are too wide apart on landing) and can only move forward by bowing out your legs. This causes excessive lateral movement. With each wide landing like this your hips (general center of mass) have to adjust and compensate for extended support time. This makes your IT band angry.

Corrective

Do five sets of ten reps of the forward change of support drill (p. 131) to execute hip movement forward.

PLANTAR FASCIITIS

Again, landing ahead of your body and a rigid (tense) ankle and foot are the root cause of this rampant injury. For plantar fasciitis this has four variations:

- Heel strike followed by neutral strike pattern that causes foot slapping and tension of the foot
- Midfoot strike with a tensed foot
- Tense active landing—tensing toes and cupping foot, and actively forcing it down
- Shoes that are too small, forcing foot into that cramped position

Corrective

1. Complete all three body weight perception drills—springiness position, running in place, and the running Pose described in Lessons One and Two (pp. 86–87, 92).

2. Jump rope for one minute and work up to three minutes, focusing on rhythm and reinforcing a proper landing pattern on the balls of your feet.

SHIN SPLINTS

Landing ahead of your body is again the culprit, causing the lower leg to land at an angle, instead of perpendicular to the ground (this also causes stress fractures and compartment syndrome). This creates a shearing effect on the shaft of the tibia bone when load is applied. Joints are designed to accept and unload, not accept and hold. Also there is an impact during active landing, which produces a shaking effect and leads to a separation of the periosteum tissues from the bone.

Corrective

Complete ten reps of the pony and change of support drills (p. 105), resting thirty seconds between each. The idea is to wire your body for landing with your foot under your hip without loading of the tibia.

LOW BACK PAIN

Landing with the foot out ahead of the body is, once again, the main cause. The lower back suffers when you compensate for this landing by bending forward with your upper body, instead of keeping your torso in a vertical position.

Corrective

Complete five reps of wall-fall drill 2 (p. 126) from the springiness position, and five reps on each leg from the running Pose. Focus on falling from your lower body, keeping your upper body aligned vertically throughout the fall.

ACHILLES TENDONITIS

This is most often caused by landing with the ankle joint locked so the heel is not allowed to touch the ground. This puts the Achilles in a stressed position and can't lengthen to absorb the impact. The other cause is pushing off the foot to create forward motion. Both of these technique issues create opposing forces, which do not allow the Achilles to lengthen properly and unload. This also has effects up the chain. Your Achilles is your first line of defense for absorbing impact that then ripples out through the rest of your body. If it can't accept the load, the rest of the body suffers.

Corrective

1. Jump rope on one or two legs at a cadence of 3 jumps per second or 180 jumps per minute. Three to five sets of thirty seconds to one minute in length.

2. Pony drill with the forward movement. Three to five sets of twenty meters at a time.

3. Go for a light run of one to three minutes in length. Three to five sets with the focus on relaxing the ankles and allowing the heels to kiss the floor after landing on the ball of the foot.

WHEN CORRECTIVES DON'T WORK

Of course, it's important to take into account the level of pain you are feeling. If you don't experience a high level of pain, then you can likely correct the problem before it worsens into a stress fracture, worn-down cartilage, or tearing of a muscle or tendon. If your level of pain is high, however, then you should refrain from all running exercises altogether so that you don't aggravate the injury.

Also, always remember to start slowly and build up. If you're struggling with a workout or a drill sequence, don't push it! Remember, an injury is not simply a setback, it's an opportunity to correct a technique flaw, adjust your pacing, and become a better runner.

PART FOUR

TAKE IT TO THE LIMIT

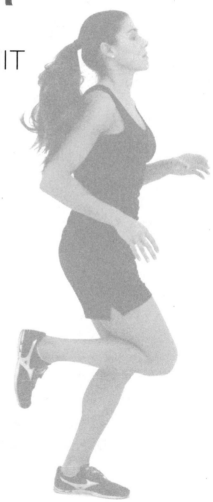

BIG MONKEY, SMALL MONKEY

How to Gauge Your Body's Training Needs

Programming a workout routine is always tricky. It's a paradox. It's supposed to be for the individual, yet it's always based on certain principles that are allegedly universally true. Ultimately, you are responsible for listening to your body and knowing what is best for you on any given day. Granted, you won't be right every time, but this part of the book will increase your odds and help you make the right decisions.

For almost fifty years, from the end of the 1920s, in my home country of Russia, a team of scientists conducted on a landmark study of the spontaneous energy activity of mammals. Let's call it Big Monkey, Small Monkey. In this study, monkeys were placed in large cages where they could move about, climb, and do a variety of activities and actions. These movements could be counted and charted. As the scientists collected baseline data regarding what constituted normal activity for each individual monkey, it became clear that some of the monkeys moved more than others. In stage two of the experiment, these same monkeys were placed in restricted cages where they couldn't move for half a day. Then they were released back to the big cages for the second half of the day. What the researchers discovered was that all of the monkeys compensated during the second half of the day to achieve their normal baseline of activity—whether high, medium, or low—for a twenty-four-hour period. Further experiments, in which individual activity quotas were deprived or exceeded, yielded similar results. For example, depriving a monkey of his or her usual activity for half a week resulted in increased activity during the second half of the week, such that the week's activity matched the individual monkey's baseline energy expenditure for a normal week. When researchers intentionally added movements above a monkey's weekly spontaneous activity, up to two times their average level, the opposite happened: The monkey reduced its activity the following week—a simian vacation that allowed the monkey to compensate for its individual "overloading" the previous week.

This experiment is significant to human sports training for obvious reasons. When designing a training program, it is essential to know if you are a big energy monkey, an average energy monkey, or a small energy monkey. This has nothing to do with your size. A big-boned, thick-muscled athlete may be more likely to be a small energy monkey and a lean, wiry athlete of average height may turn out to be a big energy monkey.

During my PhD study, I was a student of Vladimir Dijachkov's, the outstanding Soviet coach who had trained the world record holder and Olympic champion Valeri Brumel. I had access to Brumel's training logs for when he set all his world records between 1960 and 1964.

I found in these training diaries that being a small monkey, as Brumel was, didn't affect his brilliant performances. The great revelation was seeing that when he increased his training volume from three to four days a week to five to six days, his condition and performance went down.

Flash forward to the groundbreaking research done by one of America's greatest exercise physiologists, Dr. David Costill. His work has revealed that VO_2 max (your ability to efficiently consume oxygen for activity) can be improved by only 10 to 15 percent from the initial point of training. Furthermore, it takes about twelve weeks to get to this level, from which it reaches a plateau in spite of continuous training. In other words, your VO_2 max peaks. Neither a higher volume nor an increased intensity of training can raise your VO_2 max above the threshold you were born with.

So the question is: How do you figure out what kind of monkey you are? Determining which category you fit into is largely a matter of trial and error. It requires that you get in touch with how you feel physically and psychologically. If you're not matching your training to your genetic predisposition, the consequences will likely show up in your training journal in the form of inexplicable frustration, hypercriticism, and measurably decreased performance times. In all likelihood you're training too hard and need to pull back. On the other hand, if you suspect you're in the 15 percent of the population that needs to work out every single day at high volume, try ramping up your training intensity a notch. If your mood improves, you're probably a big energy monkey.

Once you've got a sense of your training disposition, you'll be ready to learn how to build a program. The four basic factors to consider are: volume, intensity, variety, and rest.

- **Volume:** How many miles are you logging a week? How many days are you training a week? How many weeks have you maintained this level of exercise? All physical activity should apply—including playing in a basketball league, lifting weights, or taking that weekly spin class.
- **Intensity:** How fast are you running—how close to your maximum speed? Sprinting is high intensity. A slow jog would be a low intensity workout.
- **Variety:** How often do you vary your workout? Do you do the same thing every day? Do you switch your workout every day? Do you switch your workout purposefully for a desired goal? Variety should be planned, not simply random.
- **Rest:** At its most basic level, rest just means time off so you can recuperate. It is your tool to prevent overtraining. As with variety, it should be planned.

These four components work together like an orchestra. Here are some general guidelines to have them work in harmony.

You should never increase volume and intensity together—that's a recipe for overtraining. If you are on a program that consistently increases volume and intensity at the same time, the body will eventually break down. It can't handle this stress for extended periods.

Variety should be applied with purpose, over the length of a training cycle—whether that's a week, a month, three months, six months, or a year. How you map out the year will depend on your personal goals, fitness level, races you might want to peak for, or distances you want to tackle.

Let's look at a one-week window. Let's say on Monday you do speed work, which is high intensity; on Wednesday you do a low intensity day for distance; and on Saturday you do a trail run or run on the beach. This would be an example of a lot of variety within a week. Taking a longer view, you could also do a four-week cycle concentrating on speed work three times a week. This means every workout would focus on speed (no endurance sessions). It all depends on your goals.

Now let's look at rest as a key part of your big picture as a runner. Pro athletes have an off-season, but many recreational runners push it year round. You need to take a chunk of time off every year. This is where the word "transition" comes into play within the rest concept. Transition means giving your body a chance to repair so you can go to the next level in performance. A transition period could be three to four weeks. It doesn't mean you become a couch potato. It means you switch up your workout and give yourself a mental break, too. You could do yoga for a month or ride a stationary bike while you read that book you've been wanting to dive into. Maybe you also get a couple of massages. Toward the end of this transition period, start to plan your next training cycle.

These are your basic tools. As a way to apply these concepts, sketch out your ideal year of training, including your monthlong transition period.

You can also use these principles to evaluate a program from a book, magazine, or Internet site that you're getting ready to start.

And don't forget to take into account what kind of monkey you are.

TRAINING PROGRAMS FOR

5K, 10K, Half Marathon, Marathon

Training, at first glance, looks like a straightforward schedule of workouts to develop a new level of running capacity. And this is true, but it is also about developing your confidence and perception. A training program builds your confidence step-by-step. It's a process of discovering how your mind and body are handling the load. In a well-designed program you learn to recognize your fatigue threshold, improve focus, and keep negative thoughts at bay.

At the heart of any training program are measurables. Measurables are data points you use to document your progress, evaluate your methods, and prevent overtraining. They track your running speed for a given workout, your distance covered at various speeds, and the number of miles you've clocked.

Each training program below requires that you train at least three times a week. The training sessions should have three parts: warm-up, main workout, and strength work—and of course you should be keeping your running journal up-to-date throughout. Each week will include a variety of times and distances, and include speed work.

Training at different speeds works all your major energy systems. You need to train through all your gears, just like a car needs to get out on the open road and move at its top speed, clearing out the cobwebs. This tunes up and conditions your athletic engine for optimal performance. To achieve your goals, this is more important than just progressively adding distance to your weekly training program. A 100-mile week does not mean you're ready for a peak marathon performance. It will more likely mean that you are marathon-miserable or marathon-injured.

Studies show that high-mileage training has limited physiological benefits after a certain point. Fitness pioneer Dr. Kenneth Cooper was the first to confirm this in his research. I have used his work and my own research over the past thirty years to create programming designed to give you the physiological foundation for each race length without unnecessary high mileage training, which creates unnecessary wear and tear on the body. The only benefit of a high mileage workout is mental. It gives you the confidence that you can complete a long race. Once you have a few long distance races under your belt, the confidence will be there and your focus can be on personal records.

The first four-week block prepares you for the 5K; each block then progressively builds on the previous block to guide you all the way to a marathon. It works like this: If you just want to run a 5K, you complete the first four-week cycle. If you want to run a 10K, you move on to the next four-week cycle. This progression continues for the longer races: For the half marathon you continue to the next four-week cycle (a twelve-week training program), and for a marathon you push on to the last four-week cycle (making your total marathon training time sixteen weeks).

If you're schedule averse and want to wing it instead, here are three simple guidelines to help you get the most out of your winging-it experience. Again, you'll need to be running a minimum of three times a week, and you should continue to complete the mobility and strength routines you've been doing all along.

1. Distance Day: On this day you run your longest distance (or for the most time). Run it at your feel good pace and enjoy it.

2. Interval Day: Run at your feel good pace, then when you feel like it pick up your pace until you are winded, then go back to a feel good pace until you recover. Try to repeat this three to five times during your run. On this day you run less distance than on your distance day.

3. Sprint Work: During your run on this day do some sprint work. You can do it before, in the middle of, or at the end of a short jogging workout (a ten-to-fifteen-minute jog at your feel good pace). Don't rest long enough to completely recover. Push yourself. Try to work up to ten sprints of around forty meters. Total running time for this day is less than your interval day.

You will have to tailor the total volume of your workouts to the length of the race you are training for. Also, try to refrain from training every day, even if you are just winging it.

THE RACES: 5K, 10K, HALF MARATHON, MARATHON

The training schedules below require you to run a minimum of three times a week. Of course, since most of us have energy thresholds large enough to sustain more frequent activity, you should expect to add an additional day or two of running or cross-training to your weekly schedule. Just make sure it's an easy run—no sprints, fartleks, or tempo runs allowed on the extra running days.

Most important, you must complete your mobility and strength routines as faithfully as you have every stage of the program leading to this moment. Now that you'll be clocking some serious mileage, these routines are more important than ever. The same goes for your running journal. With increased distance comes the increased likelihood that technique flaws will lead to injury. Documenting your workouts will enable you to detect problems before they get out of control. You need to be especially mindful of your technique when fatigue sets in. Your journal is a way to track consciously what often happens unconsciously. If you're not aware of technique issues, you can't fix them.

The same goes for filming. All the elements in this program work together as an integrated system. Continue to capture and analyze yourself on video periodically throughout your training program. The asterisks in the schedules below denote optimum moments to videotape your running form.

How to Use the Race Ready Chart

The race ready training program is designed to take your training to the next level after you've completed the ten lessons and the nine-week running circuit. Here are the basic guidelines:

- If the workouts for week one of the program are too difficult, start with a time and a distance you are comfortable with and work up to the week one goals.
- During speed days, if the workout is too difficult, take a longer rest between each run or cut down the number of repetitions for each run. In general, you should rest for ninety seconds between runs or until you get your breath back.

- To avoid confusing fractions and keep the numbers simple, the distances are measured in a familiar mix of miles and kilometers.
- The program was designed for a mid-level runner. Charts for different levels, from beginner to advanced, can be downloaded at posemethod.com.

Remember, it's always about quality over quantity. You still have to stay vigilant to master a new technique. All of this has the same set of goals that we discussed from the start: running faster, farther, and injury-free for life.

Race	Week	Day One	Day Two	Day Three
5K, 10K, HALF MARATHON, MARATHON	1*	5 miles (47–50 minutes) 5 × 200 meters (48–51 seconds)	1K (4:35–4:54 minutes) 5 × 800 meters (4:06– 4:22 minutes) 400 meters (1:40–1:46)	2K (9:23–10:00 minutes)
	2	10K (56:40–60:00 minutes) 5 × 200 meters (48–50 seconds)	400 meters (1:40–1:46 minutes) 10-minute easy jog 2 × 1K (4:35–4:54 minutes) 2 × 600 meters (2:40–2:46 minutes)	30-minute easy jog 2 × 3K (14:06–15:05 minutes)
	3*	10K (56:40– 60:00 minutes) 5 × 200 meters (48–50 seconds)	400 meters (1:40–1:46 minutes) 10-minute easy jog 2 × 1K (4:35–4:54 minutes) 2 × 600 meters (2:40–2:46 minutes)	30-minute easy jog 3K (13:40–14:38 minutes) 2k (8:53–9:30 minutes)
	4	30-minute easy jog	20-minute easy jog 5 × 200 meters (48–50 seconds)	**5K Race**
10K, HALF MARATHON, MARATHON	5*	2K (9:58–10:45 minutes) 1K (4:47–5:06 minutes) 600 meters (2:50–3:02 minutes) 400 meters (1:39–1:46 minutes)	10 miles (1:43–1:48 hours) 5 × 200 meters (49–50 seconds)	10K (53:20–57:00 minutes)
	6	2 × 2K (9:23–10:00 minutes) 2 × 1K (4:40–4:58 minutes) 600 meters (2:40–2:51 minutes) 400 meters (1:34–1:40 minutes)	Half marathon (2:09–2:16 hours) 5 × 200 meters (48–50 seconds)	10K (51:20–54:45 minutes)

Race	Week	Day One	Day Two	Day Three
	7	2K (9:10–9:48 minutes) 1K (4:20–4:38 minutes)	8 miles (1:22–1:26 hours) 3 × 200 meters (47–50 seconds)	10K (50:14–53:36 minutes)
	8	2 × 600 meters (2:50–3:00 minutes) 2 × 400 meters (1:36–1:42 minutes)	5-minute easy jog 5 × 200 meters (47–50 seconds)	**10K Race**
HALF MARATHON, MARATHON	9*	1 mile (7:50–8:36 minutes) 800 meters (4:16–4:32 minutes) 600 meters (2:51–3:03 minutes)	2 × 400 meters (1:45–1:52 minutes) 5K (27:16–29:10 minutes)	10 miles (1:29–1:31 hours) 5 × 200 meters (47–51 seconds)
	10	2 × 1 mile (7:46–8:18 minutes) 2 × 800 meters (4:17–4:22 minutes)	2 × 5K (27:16–29:10 minutes) 2 × 400 meters (1:40–1:46 minutes)	Half Marathon (1:54–2:00 hours) 5 × 200 meters (47–51 seconds)
	11*	1 mile (7:10–7:38 minutes) 800 meters (3:51–4:07 minutes) 600 meters (2:36–2:47 minutes)	5K (25:39–27:23 minutes) 3 × 400 meters (1:34–1:40 minutes)	10 miles (1:27–1:29 hours) 5 × 200 meters (46–48 seconds)
	12	2 × 600 meters (2:50–3:00 minutes) 2 × 400 meters (1:36–1:42 minutes)	5-minute easy jog 5 × 200 meters (47–50 seconds)	**Half Marathon**
MARATHON	13*	10K (56–60 minutes)	2 × 2K (9:58–10:42 minutes) 600 meters (2:46–2:58 minutes) 400 meters (1:46–1:50 minutes)	Half marathon (2:00–2:06 hours) 5 × 200 meters (48–50 seconds)
	14	2-hour easy run 2 × 3K (15:06–16:03 minutes)	10K (53:20–57:00 minutes) 600 meters (2:46–2:58 minutes) 400 meters (1:40–1:46 minutes)	Half marathon (1:57–2:03 hours) 5 × 200 meters (48–50 seconds)
	15	1-hour easy run 2K (9:23–10:00 minutes) 600 meters (2:36–2:47 minutes)	1-hour easy run 600 meters (2:52–3:08 minutes) 400 meters (1:43–1:50 minutes)	10 miles (1:29–1:33 hours) 5 × 200 meters (47–49 seconds)
	16	10K (1:00–1:04 hours)	5 × 200 meters (easy pace)	**Marathon**
*Video Capture				

RUNNING FOR A LIFETIME

Staying Healthy, Having Fun, Personal Records

So you've made it through the program, maybe even run a few races. But this is just the first step. The nuances and rewards of running are every bit as complicated as the famously lifelong sports of golf and tennis. Just as golfers spend their whole lives working on their swings and still have good days and bad days on the course, you'll be constantly evaluating and perfecting your form, enjoying days when running is effortless and soldiering through days when it's a challenge. The important thing is that now you have the tools and techniques for a lifetime of running. If you love running, why not be the best runner you can be?

Keep creating your next set of goals. If you achieved a personal record in the 10K last month, consider training for a marathon. But also remember to build up gradually. Always start again at week one so that you don't overload yourself with too much volume at once—the speed of your sprints and intervals will obviously increase the more you train, but your perceived effort should remain steady. It's essential that you keep up with your movement preparation and strength routines, just as it's essential that you continue to analyze your form on film and keep a detailed running journal. As the months and years accrue, you'll have the pleasure of looking back on your observations, seeing how patterns of exertion, recovery, and refined technique emerge over a lifetime of running. Today, next year, a decade from now, you are a mindful runner always honing your perception, always striving to hit that perfect stride over and over again.

APPENDIX

Cheat Sheet

RULES OF GOOD RUNNING TECHNIQUE

1. Free-fall by moving your hips (general center of mass) over your point of support (the balls of your feet).

2. Keep shoulders, hips and ankles in proper Pose alignment.

3. Always keep your knees bent; don't straighten them.

4. Keep your body weight on balls of your feet.

5. Change support quickly from one foot to the other.

6. Pull the ankle from the ground straight up under the hip.

7. Make your time on support short.

8. Don't push off your foot or drive your knee, trying to use thigh and quad muscles to drive you forward, instead of harnessing the power of gravity.

9. Don't land on the heels or put weight on your heels while on support. Your heels should only lightly touch the ground.

10. Falling starts when the heel of your support foot comes off the ground.

11. Falling ends when the foot of your swing leg passes the knee of your support leg.

12. Don't try to increase your stride or range of motion to increase your speed.

13. Don't fixate on landing. Focus on pulling.

14. Your legs should land effortlessly without any muscle activity,

15. Keep your feet in a neutral position.

16. Arms act as a counterbalance to the legs.

COMMON ERRORS IN RUNNING

1. Landing with the heel first.

2. Landing ahead of the body—overstriding.

3. Using quad muscles (push off) instead of the hamstring to pull your foot off the ground.

4. Landing on the toes in front of your hips (your general center of mass).

5. Don't reach with the toes—known as plantar flexion.

6. Actively landing on your forefoot.

7. Too much muscle tension in parts of the body that aren't doing the primary work.

8. Pulling late.

9. Keeping shoulders stiff and not unloading.

10. Pumping arms.

11. Wrong thinking, not giving yourself the proper commands.

12. Wrong images, not being able to see the proper technique in your mind's eye.

UNITED STATES ARMY ASSESSMENT

I developed the following training assessment for the U. S. Army to give soldiers a snapshot of what their times would be for different race distances. This same system will work for you. The first step is to time yourself in a 400-meter run at your top speed. A quick word of caution: this is just a test. You have created a fitness foundation with your nine-week circuit, but err on the side of safety and use common sense when pushing yourself on this test. Your top speed should feel safe, and you shouldn't feel like you're going to pass out at the end of the test. Also, make sure you are properly warmed up. Your 400-meter time becomes the benchmark for predicting your race times in the chart below. This will give you a sense of where you are and help you set practical goals.

MARATHON	2:30.0	2:45.0	3:00.0	3:15.0	3:30.0
400M	56.0–59.0	61.0–64.0	1:07.0–1:10.0	1:13.0–1:16.0	1:18.0–1:21.0

HALF MARATHON	1:20.0	1:30.0	1:40.0	1:50.0	2:00.0
400M	60.0–63.0	1:07.0–1:10.0	1:15.0–1:18.0	1:22.0–1:25.0	1:30.0–1:33.0

10KM	35:00	40:00	45:00	50:00	55:00
400M	1:02.0–1:05.0	1:10.0–1:13.0	1:19.0–1:22.0	1:27.0–1:30.0	1:36.0–1:39.0

5KM	18:00	21:00	24:00	27:00	30:00
400M	1:03.0–1:06.0	1:13.0–1:16.0	1:24.0–1:27.0	1:34.0–1:37.0	1:45.0–1:48.0

Table of interrelations of 400-meter time with different race distances.

ANATOMY OF A STRIDE

Heel	Midfoot	Forefoot	Paw Back
Joints Absorb Impact	Excess Strain on Knee	Minimal Joint Strain	Physically Impossible

Heel	Midfoot	Forefoot	Paw Back
- Locked ankle, knee, and hip joints - Impact: absorb up to 3x body weight every stride - Longest support time -Suppination and pronation	-Braking effect: ahead of the body every time -Leverage on the knee: produces excess strain -Flat-foot landing: hard to consistently reproduce -Anatomically impossible to land on the arch	-Unlocked: impact redistributed -Minimal braking effect and joint strain -Shortest support time -Maximum elasticity	-Body weight is behind the foot -We lack the strength and force to produce rotational movement of the body -When the body weight is not available the muscles do not work

Here's a visual cheat sheet with notes on running optimally.

nning Pose
otimal Balance

-refoot to Pose is the
ost efficient transfer
the body forward
cilitates acceleration
a rotation
alanced alignment of
ead, shoulders, hips
d feet
asticity: S-like body

Falling
Running Faster

Invariable

-The degree of falling
 forward determines your
 running speed
-Falling in the Pose
 position is the most
 efficient way to
 accelerate
-Pumping of arms does
 not directly contribute
 to forward movement

Knee Drive
Slows You Down

-Over emphasizes use of
 hip flexors
-Slows down the general
 center of mass to
 compensate for the
 swing leg moving
 forward

Push Off
Wasted Energy

-Pushing off is mostly
 possible only in the
 vertical direction,
 increasing our vertical
 oscillation but providing
 little horizontal
 movement
-The ankle is the slowest
 joint in our body and
 only 2% of our body
 weight

Pulling
Running Longer

Invariable

-On average, runners must
 increase cadence by 15
 spm to begin to utilize
 muscle-tendon elasticity
-Mechanical efficiency
 can increase running
 economy
-Magnitude of the pulling
 action is determined by
 the angle of falling

6-POINT RUNNING ANALYSIS

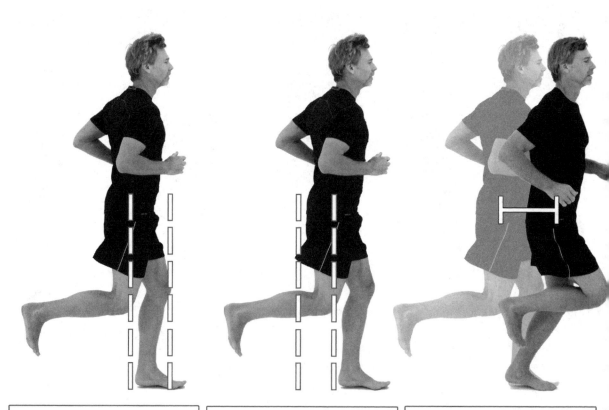

1 - Initial Contact	2 - Trail Leg Distance	3 - Frame Count to Pose
Foot hits in slight suppination as close to directly under the body as possible	The trail leg is only slightly behind the body at initial contact	It takes one frame for the body to arrive at the running Pose

Here's a visual cheat sheet with notes on running optimally.

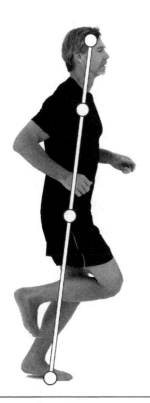

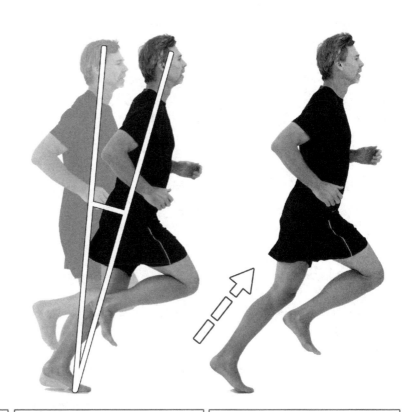

4 - Pose Alignment

The body alignment in the running Pose is close to completely vertical

5 - Fall Threshold

From the vertical, fall until the foot of the swing leg passes the support knee

6 - Frame Count to Pull

It takes one frame to go from the running Pose to initiate Pulling

GLOSSARY

angle of falling

Speed relates to your angle of falling. Imagine you are balancing one of those long foam rollers on your fingertips. As it falls forward, you move your hand directly underneath it to bring it back to its upright position. The farther it falls forward—the more extreme the angle—the more difficult it is to get your hand underneath to bring it back to the upright position. Once the foam roll passes a certain angle it's impossible to get your hand underneath in time and it falls to the ground. It's the same with running: The farther your body falls forward the faster you have to bring your swing leg through to catch yourself in the Pose stance. When you run, you don't fall like the foam roller, uniformly from top to bottom; you fall from your hips or the center of your body. Your torso stays upright and doesn't lean. This is a concept you'll understand better through doing.

body weight

The manifestation of gravitational force that pulls any mass toward the ground. Body weight is directly related to support. You determine how you are applying your body weight by where you feel the most pressure. For example, if you feel the most pressure on the balls of your feet, then that's where you are applying your body weight. If you feel most of the pressure on your heels, then you're applying body weight to your heels.

cadence

Cadence is the number of steps taken in a set time, usually per minute.

center of gravity

Your body's center of gravity is the point of application of the resultant force of gravity acting on separate parts of the body. It also changes depending on your activity. But as a working definition, when you are standing in your springiness position your center of gravity will be about two inches below your belly button.

flight phase

This occurs when both feet are off the ground during running. In traditional terminology this is also called the recovery phase.

geometric restraint

This is your body's natural protective mechanism that slows down movement as a joint gets close to full extension. The body does this to avoid injury (like hyperextension). If you look at footage of top runners, they never fully extend their legs during running. This would only slow them down and increase the chance of injury.

gravity

Gravity affects every body and every object on the planet the same way. This in turn affects the way you move and run. There is only one optimal way to run and that is to harness the gift of gravity. To take advantage of gravity, you move your hips forward past your support foot, letting your body catch the wind of gravity, propelling you forward.

ground reaction force (GRF)

Ground reaction force happens when your foot makes contact with the ground. The impact of the foot making contact with the ground initiates the ground pushing back with equal force. This is an example of Newton's Third Law: For every reaction there is an equal and opposite reaction. GRF doesn't move you forward—it's just a reaction. The science community has formed an agreement on this matter.

landing (contact and support)

In Pose you want to land on the ball of your foot under your hip. You want the contact to be quick and quiet. You want to avoid landing on your heel first with your foot well ahead of your hips. This doesn't mean the heel shouldn't touch the ground at all. You want the heel to touch the ground with a little kiss. The main thing to remember about landing is that most of your body weight should be on the ball of your foot.

muscle-tendon elasticity in running

Muscle-tendon elasticity is how the body handles the impact of running and turns a negative into a positive. When your foot makes contact with the ground, your muscles and tendons lengthen and absorb the impact. The muscles and tendons then shorten, releasing the absorbed energy back into the running movement while the body weight leaves from support. A simple example is the action of a bow and arrow. Pulling the bowstring back is like lengthening and loading the muscle. Releasing the bowstring (letting the arrow fly) is like the tendon shortening and releasing energy back into the stride.

This is more accurately described as a muscle-tendon elasticity system—it includes tendons and ligaments, like a shock absorber spring and its attachments. The entire system stores and releases energy.

In the world of exercise science this is also called the stretch-shortening cycle. When the muscle-tendon system is effectively used, the energy cost of running can be reduced by 50 percent. In short, you will use less energy and perform better when you don't over-muscle your stride.

overstride

A classic overstride is when your foot lands out in front of your body, instead of under your hip.

Pose core

From your center of gravity in outward ripples is your core, or your power center, also called your pillar strength, or your powerhouse. The core now has so many names that it can be confusing. This is more than just your abs. It's your abs, back, and glute muscles; your hips, your lower back, your shoulder girdle, and your spine. The Pose core is a little different from the traditional core because it relates to running, so it includes your whole spine.

For running, if you drew a box around your body it would start just below your butt and go all the way up to your shoulders. Your head floats naturally on top of this. The force and movement of running will be transferred most efficiently in a straight line through an aligned body. When you have weak links that drift out of alignment because of weak muscles or mobility or stability issues in your joints, you will not run as efficiently.

Pose position alignment

The line of support that runs from the ball of your foot through your hip, shoulder, and ear. This alignment is essential for harnessing the potential energy of falling, using gravity, and utilizing muscle-tendon elasticity.

pull magnitude

How high you bring your pull leg toward your butt in your running stride. This is related to how fast you're running. The faster you run, the greater your pull magnitude (heel closer to your butt); the slower, the less your magnitude (heel farther away from your butt). In a jog your heel won't even go above your knee.

running

Running requires that both feet have to be off the ground at some point in your stride, otherwise you would be walking.

S-shape curve

This is the shape the body assumes during running: The body never fully extends its joints, but maintains the S-like coiled spring posture (just like the fastest animals) during running, taking full advantage of muscle-tendon elasticity and geometric restraint.

springiness position

Springiness position is a position of readiness for movement. You are on the balls of your feet and in proper Pose alignment. For a more detailed description go to p. 13. You should become familiar with this position before you start exercising or doing any of the lessons.

step

The time between the contact of one foot with the ground and the contact of the next foot.

stride

The time between the contact of one foot with the ground and the subsequent contact of the same foot.

stride length

The distance between your previous support and upcoming landing.

swing leg

The airborne leg that moves past the support leg in the flight phase, then lands and becomes the new support leg.

torque

The rotational effect of a force on an object. In the runner's case, the downward pull of gravity is the force, while the runner's center of mass rotates forward on the support leg to move the runner forward.

walking

Walking is defined as having one support foot on the ground at all times.

DRILL INDEX

INDEX

Page numbers in *italics* refer to illustrations.